Fit and Fabulous After 40

ALSO BY DENISE AUSTIN

Lose Those Last 10 Pounds

JumpStart

Hit the Spot!

Denise Austin's Ultimate Pregnancy Book

Fit and Fabulous
After 40

*A 5-Part Program for
Turning Back the Clock*

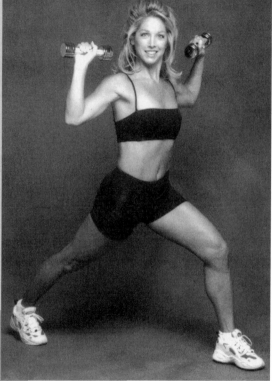

Denise Austin

BROADWAY BOOKS *New York*

BROADWAY

FIT AND FABULOUS AFTER 40. Copyright © 2001 by Denise Austin. All
rights reserved. Printed in the United States of America. No part of this book
may be reproduced or transmitted in any form or by any means, electronic
or mechanical, including photocopying, recording, or by any information
storage and retrieval system, without written permission from the publisher.
For information, address Broadway Books, a division of Random House, Inc.,
1540 Broadway, New York, NY 10036.

Broadway Books titles may be purchased for business or promotional use or for
special sales. For information, please write to: Special Markets Department,
Random House, Inc., 1540 Broadway, New York, NY 10036.

BROADWAY BOOKS and its logo, a letter B bisected on the diagonal, are
trademarks of Broadway Books, a division of Random House, Inc.

Visit our Web site at www.broadwaybooks.com

Library of Congress Cataloging-in-Publication Data
Austin, Denise.
    Fit and fabulous after 40 : a 5-part program for turning back the clock /
    Denise Austin.—1st ed.
        p. cm.
    ISBN 0-7679-0471-0
    1. Exercise for women. 2. Physical fitness for women. 3. Middle aged
women—Health and hygiene. 4. Physical fitness for middle aged persons.
    I. Title: Fit and fabulous after forty. II. Title.

RA778 .A8755 2001
613.7'045—dc21

00-050714

FIRST EDITION

Designed by Erin L. Matherne and Tina Thompson

01 02 03 04 10 9 8 7 6 5 4 3 2 1

Disclaimer

The instructions and advice in this book are in no way intended as a substitute for medical counseling. We advise the reader to consult with his/her doctor before beginning this or any diet and regimen of exercise. The author and the publisher disclaim any liability or loss, personal or otherwise, resulting from the procedures in this book.

To my Mom who was and always will be the center of my life. . . .
Her enthusiasm for life, her laughter and mostly her unflagging love
and devotion to her children and grandchildren remain an inspiration.

My Mom's love and encouragement will stay with me
and my children throughout our lives.

Acknowledgments

When it comes to thanking people, I always think of my mom first. I have just experienced the loss of my mother, my best friend. My cute little mom passed away on November 2, 2000 (All Soul's Day) peacefully at home with all four of her daughters by her side. Mom was so fun, vital and full of life until the day just four months ago when we found out she had a brain tumor. This was a form of cancer that had nothing to do with lifestyle. She did everything right her whole life—never smoked or drank, ate well, was active and had a terrific positive attitude. But God needed her in Heaven. I will miss her terribly, but the memories will live forever.

To my husband, Jeff, who has given me so much love and support. Thank you honey-bunny! To my daughters, Kelly and Katie, my most precious gifts from God. I love being a mom.

To my brother, Michael Katnich, and my sisters: Kristine Kelly, Anne Giltner and Donna Boucher. We are all so blessed to have such a close bond. We love to be around one another; we laugh so hard together.

I want to thank Stacy and Wynne Whitman (sisters), along with Dale Burg, for their research and contributions to this book.

A big thanks to my dear friend Stephanie Mansfield for "shaping up" this book and just being there when I needed her the most.

Thanks to Leslie Bonci, R.D., and Edith Howard Hogan, R.D., the two top nutritionists in the country. Also, to Olivia Sheldon for her yoga expertise.

A special thanks to Marc Haines, a great chef in Dallas, Texas, for his delicious recipes.

Many thanks to my editor, Ann Campbell, and her assistant, Amanda Gross, for all their help, and to Jan Miller, the best literary agent ever.

And to all my friends who continue to show their support and true friendship; I love you all. Thank you.

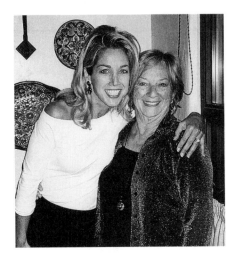

Me and my Mom

Contents

Introduction

The invitation arrives in the mail.

Your first reaction? *Panic.*

It might be a high school reunion or wedding, a graduation or anniversary black-tie gala. Suddenly you feel self-conscious. It's been months since you found the time to fit exercise into your daily schedule and that little black dress is two sizes too small. "How will I measure up?" you worry. "Do I look older than my friends?"

Some of my best friends—sharp, wise and wonderful women— all say they share the same concerns, especially once they hit 40. They have strange appetite cravings. They feel fatigued. Their waistlines are expanding. Almost overnight, nothing seems to fit. Their metabolism has screeched to a halt. The thought of eating even one brownie translates into an hour on the treadmill.

"Denise, how do you do it?" they ask. "How do you manage to stay so fit and look so young?"

In this book I want to share the answer with you.

The truth, however tough it might be for us to admit, is that our bodies have changed. We're different, and not just because of our evolving careers and personal lives. And while you probably feel more successful in your professional and private life now than you did in your 20s (I know I do), you are as nervous about your appearance as a teenager on the eve of the prom. Your skin may not be as supple (those freckles and brown spots! those jiggly arms!), your hair not as shiny. Your hormones have you on a roller coaster. You may find your sleep interrupted, your memory fuzzy, your moods unpredictable. The stress of maintaining a job and caring for a husband and children (and sometimes aging parents) shows in the dark crescents under your eyes.

But trust me—we are *all* going through this together. The good news is that you *can* take steps to prevent and minimize these changes, steps that can help you recapture that youthful glow and stop worrying about that upcoming high school reunion. But turning back the clock takes more than a crash diet or European facial. It's not about quick fixes anymore. It's about *real* lifestyle changes that will rejuvenate a woman in her 40s, help her gain control over the aging process and pave the way for looking fit and fabulous into her 50s, 60s and beyond.

I admire so many over-40 women: Rene Russo, Susan Sarandon, Tina Turner, Goldie Hawn, Kate Capshaw, Sela Ward and Catherine Deneuve have all shown us that real beauty is ageless. To me, they are sexier than most 20-somethings. I admire the fact that they work at it, staying fit and eating sensibly. But most important, they maintain an upbeat outlook with each passing year. They have certainly turned back Hollywood's clock!

It's important for all of us to remember that our 40s are rich in possibilities. In fact, in a study conducted by the MacArthur Foundation, researchers found that midlife was indeed the happiest time for most men and especially women, who scored higher on areas like personal growth. The groundbreaking 10-year study involved nearly 8,000 Americans between 25 and 75 and debunked the myth of the "midlife crisis." Women in particular said they felt a greater sense of control and that life was more rewarding after 40. They also said they feel nearly 15 years younger than their physical appearances!

The bad news? A majority of women, especially those 35 to 54, reported feeling more demands at home, and almost half said they were not as physically fit as they were five years ago. The older we get, the more responsibilities we seem to have, and all too often that means we don't find the time to take care of ourselves.

As a former gymnast, I've always taken care of my body. In my 20s, however, I was more concerned with looking good in a bikini (I did grow up in California, after all). These days I'm focused on feeling good and staying healthy—and if I can still get away with wearing a bikini, that's a bonus! I actively try to make healthy choices in terms of what I eat and how I treat my body—I'm careful about sunscreen, I rarely drink and I make sure that I work out almost every day, not just because it's my job, but because it's so vital to my health and well-being. Naturally, sometimes it's hard. The days seem shorter, and sometimes my schedule can be frantic. I'm often forced to eat on the run and yes, I find myself in the fast-food drive-through window trying to choose something healthy when I'm craving french fries and a milkshake.

But, like so many women out there, I had a cholesterol test last year, and my level was high—218. Fortunately, with a few changes in my diet (no more partially hydrogenated foods, french fries, potato chips or non-dairy creamer) the number went down. I'm now at 170. Although I'm in good health overall, it is a worry, especially as I get older. For me, it was the first real flag to signal that my body is changing—that I need to pay more attention to what I eat if I want to remain in peak physical condition and avoid bigger problems down the road.

One of the benefits of aging is appreciating good health. I feel lucky to have been blessed with two pregnancies with no complications, and I'm religious about yearly checkups. But I'm definitely a realist. I know certain health problems can crop up (a friend of mine was recently diagnosed with breast cancer) and I'm not afraid of facing them if and when they do. That's part of life. But since turning 40 I feel stronger about my priorities: being happy and healthy, spending time with those I love and working with people I enjoy. When filming my television show, I work with the same wonderful people who have been with me for years. They make a big difference in how I feel, especially in front of the camera. They are truly like family to me. And no matter how busy I am, I try to check in with my friends on a regular basis (I seem to spend half my time in television green rooms gabbing to my friends on the phone). I talk to my three sisters, who live in California, just about every day. After 17 years of marriage my husband, Jeff, and I have an enduring relationship, based on love, laughter, respect and mutual admiration. He's the best! And so are my two beautiful daughters, Kelly and Katie. Being a mom is my greatest achievement and I hope that my girls continue to grow and thrive with their boundless joy and energy.

Some women view aging with despair, while some adopt a certain bravado. I'll never forget the slogan on the T-shirt Gloria Steinem wore when she celebrated her birthday: This Is What 40 Looks Like. Other women are not so confident. "Why bother taking care of myself?" they say. "The aging process is inevitable."

My answer? Every single day is a gift.

Statistics show that the average American woman can expect to live to the age of 79. My grandmother, who walked to church every morning and never had a driver's license, lived to be 94. Jeff's grandma, who read three books each week and exercised every day, lived to 102. I was amazed at how active she remained. But this means that you very likely have at least *four decades* ahead of you! And it's not too late to start preparing for what could be the most satisfying years of your life.

I won't kid you. There are certain aspects of aging that bother me. Every once in a while I look in the mirror and see tiny wrinkles and squint lines that weren't there before (Jeff always says they're my laugh lines). And then there's that droopy skin above my kneecaps or near my elbows. Where did that come from?

But the truth is that I don't really feel older than I did 20 years ago. So why should I look it? Today we have the knowledge and the means to look and feel better than our mothers did at our age. We know about the dangers of smoking and excessive drinking. We know how chronic stress can lead to heart disease and other ills. We know more about the importance of exercise and strength training to build lean muscle and stave off bone loss. We owe it to our husbands and children, and most of all to ourselves, to make the most of the coming years. To be vital and strong, to have endurance and energy. To care for ourselves as much as we care for our families and friends.

I was talking to a friend the other day and she said, "What is it about turning 40? I finally feel mentally and emotionally at peace, just at the point my body decides to rebel."

I reassured her that it *is* possible to stop or delay many of these changes—by accepting the challenge of growing older and taking control. Over the years I have learned there's only one thing I truly have power over and one thing I can always improve: myself.

YOU have the power to fight the aging process and turn back the clock! We're going to do it together, starting today, by following the program outlined in this book. You'll be amazed by the changes that take place. So get ready to embark on a new phase of your life—one that I hope will be more rewarding than anything you've experienced thus far. I'll be with you every step of the way.

People often seem surprised when they discover my age (I celebrated my 43rd birthday a few months ago), which is always flattering. I guess it means I'm doing something right. How do I manage to look so young? Where do I get my energy? How do I seem to do it all—handle a career, a family, a social life and a regular exercise program? (Confession: Unlike Martha Stewart, I need more than four hours of sleep a night, and some days I don't get out of my jammies until the kids have seconds on French toast!)

After nearly 25 years as a health and fitness professional, I have learned the secrets of staying young and vital. That's why I'm writing this book—I want to share with you everything I know and everything I believe about looking young, staying fit and feeling fabulous in your 40s. By keeping up with the latest research and interviewing the top experts in the field, I know what works and what doesn't. I know the fads from the facts. I get thousands of letters each year from women who have tried all sorts of "instant" weight-loss plans and "miracle" anti-aging remedies that are ultimately doomed to fail. I am familiar with your questions and concerns from talking to the women who come to my personal appearances and who watch my television show on Lifetime. They want my advice because they know I'll give it to them straight! Through listening to their experiences and finding the best, medically sound practices that really work, I've developed a safe, highly effective formula for staying fit and fabulous. This book shows you how to use the formula to:

- Stop the Clock with exercises to trim and shape your over-40 body
- Lose those stubborn extra pounds and NOT regain them
- Develop a stretching and strength-training plan for the rest of your life
- Benefit from my new "Nutrient Rich" diet especially designed for women over 40
- Transform your negative thinking into a positive outlook
- Learn my personal anti-aging tips, the ones that really work

The program is simple. My Anti-Aging Pyramid concentrates on five critical levels of being your best after 40: exercise, nutrition, health, beauty and mental attitude. Each of the five components is dependent on the others.

There are no crash diets, expensive wrinkle creams or magic pills. In fact, it's an all-natural, sensible approach to maintaining optimal health. You'll find tips on losing that stubborn over-40 weight safely and effectively, and understand how to keep it off. My age-defying exercises will help you build calorie-burning muscle, fight gravity, tone up so you won't "sag" and age-proof your bones. I've included the latest information on anti-aging foods and supplements as well as quick, delicious recipes for healthy home-cooked meals. (And yes, Jeff and I both love tacos, chocolate pie and the occasional beer!)

You'll also find guidelines for protecting yourself against heart disease, cancer and other diseases. You'll learn why a bone density test is just as important as a mammogram after 40. I also offer advice on how to talk frankly to your doctor about specific concerns. As a bonus, you'll also learn my favorite secrets for eliminating wrinkles and keeping your hair shiny and thick.

As you start doing the program, you'll be amazed by the results—I've seen them firsthand time and time again, both in myself and in my sisters and friends who have followed the advice presented here. It's an ongoing process, and turning back the clock requires drive and willingness on your part, but trust me—when you get up to dance at your daughter's wedding or slip into that gorgeous evening gown on your 30th anniversary, it will be well worth the effort.

Author and poet Hervey Allen wrote, "The only time you really live fully is from thirty to sixty. The young are slaves to dreams; the old servants of regrets. Only the middle-aged have all their five senses in the keeping of their wits."

So let's keep our wits, along with our waistlines!

And stay fit and fabulous *forever.*

1

The Pyramid Plan

Denise Austin's Anti-Aging Pyramid

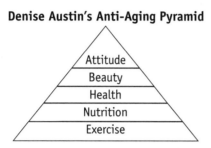

Attitude
Beauty
Health
Nutrition
Exercise

Congratulations! Just by reading these words, you've already taken an important first step toward improving your life and your health: You've made the decision to do it. But now you're not sure what to do next. You know that you need to exercise more. You definitely want to lose those love handles. And you would love to diminish your wrinkles and get rid of those brown spots on your skin. So where do you go from here? And how can you create a program that can tackle all of these different issues?

Before we delve into the program itself, let's take a closer look at the aging process and some of the major changes that women face as they grow older.

IN YOUR 40S

Maybe the kids are out of the house (at least in school during the day, like mine) and you've finally gotten a chance to sit, relax and catch up on the latest books. Or maybe you're focusing on your career and spending most of your time sitting behind a desk. Either way, you're probably not getting enough exercise.

Without regular exercise, muscles shrink at a rate of 1 to 2 percent per year. The more muscle you lose, the slower your metabolism gets and the fewer calories your body burns. If your eating habits don't change, your waistline starts to expand and your pants get tighter. You can expect to gain about 10 pounds between the ages of 40 and 50.

All that sitting around combined with a poor diet and perhaps cigarette smoking (please quit now) as well may also be causing your bones to get steadily weaker. Your muscles start to atrophy due to inactivity, and your joints (especially your knees and hips) are beginning to feel stiff and creaky.

If you haven't been taking proper care of your skin, sun damage might appear in the form of wrinkles around your eyes and on your forehead, especially now that the production of collagen—a protein found in skin tissue that gives it elasticity and firmness—has begun to slow down.

IN YOUR 50S

The average woman experiences menopause at age 51, after which estrogen levels decrease by as much as 75 percent. A decline in estrogen causes cholesterol levels to rise and blood vessels to become less elastic, putting your heart at risk. As estrogen levels plummet, bone loss becomes more rapid, upping your risk of fractures. Fat—which had previously been stored in the hips and buttocks, primarily for breast-feeding—begins to collect more in your abdomen and you develop a "pot belly."

Your skin also becomes thinner, drier and less elastic due to this drop in estrogen as well as years of sun exposure and lack of proper nutrition. Wrinkles may begin to appear at the corners of your mouth and become more prominent on other parts of your face and body. Reduced circulation may cause your once-rosy cheeks to look pale and colorless.

IN YOUR 60S

If you remain inactive, your muscles and ligaments keep getting weaker. Your joints get "rusty," and you lose your flexibility. Your weight distribution has also changed due to more fat around your middle. As a result, you lose your balance more easily.

As your muscles and bones continue to shrink, your posture may become slumped. With the exception of your pot belly, your body seems to be getting smaller. Next to you, your grown-up kids appear to be getting taller and taller.

Remember: If you don't use it, you'll lose it. If you rest, you rust.

If you've continued to neglect it, your skin becomes slacker and wrinkling increases. Skin pigmentation starts to clump in some places, causing brown spots. Due to a higher cell turnover, skin cells become irregularly shaped, and precancerous lesions are more likely.

• • •

Many of these changes result from the shifting in hormones that occurs as our bodies, no longer primed for childbearing, go through peri-menopause (the months or years immediately before our periods stop) and menopause, when they actually do. While most of our mothers sat down with us and rather awkwardly and tenderly explained menstruation, all too often the subject of menopause is overlooked. Even our doctors may be slow to advise us of this natural biological transition. But if we're going to beat the aging process, it's important to understand exactly what's going on inside our bodies and how it can affect our health and appearance—if we don't take action, that is!

For most women, this change in hormones usually begins in their 40s as we begin to lose estrogen, progesterone and testosterone. Many women barely notice the transition taking place; others experience headaches, depression and insomnia. One major side effect—and one of the first that many of us notice—is weight gain. But other studies have shown that menopause alone is rarely the culprit, and that calorie consumption and exercise habits are equally responsible for those added pounds. Experts say that after the age of 40, a woman's metabolism slows about 5 to 7 percent each decade. You may have consumed over 2,000 calories a day as a young woman, but after the age of 40 you should probably limit your caloric intake to approximately 1,700 if you want to avoid middle-age spread. This drop in metabolism is partly the result of a decrease in muscle mass—primarily due to a more sedentary lifestyle—that reduces our ability to burn calories.

My Anti-Aging Pyramid consists of five parts: exercise, nutrition, health, beauty and attitude. Each piece of the pyramid works in conjunction with the others to create an overall plan for reversing the aging process. Don't forget: Well-being is more than just exercise. It's more than just eating soy and broccoli. To be truly healthy and defy the aging process, you need balance in every aspect of your life, including your workouts, your diet, your job, your relationships and your outlook on life.

To better explain, I'll use one of my favorite analogies. Your body is like a sophisticated machine—think of it as a Mercedes. If the gas tank is empty, the brakes are shot or one tire is flat, that car is going to sit in the driveway, eventually getting old and rusty. In neglecting to tend to a single problem, you eventually lose the entire machine. Similarly, if you approach your day with negative thoughts, grumbling about your hectic schedule or the lousy weather, chances are you'll lack the incentive to eat well and hit the gym, which in turn can put you in an even worse mood and leave your stress levels soaring as you count up your calories at the end of the day and worry about fitting into that new dress you bought. It's all connected.

Throughout the book I'll talk about each section of the pyramid separately, starting at the bottom and working our way up. Since each building block is interconnected, you may notice some overlap. For instance, water is essential to keep you hydrated while working out, but it's also vital for beautiful skin and hair. So you'll find references to drinking water in both the exercise and beauty departments.

I've specifically placed exercise and diet at the base of my Anti-Aging Pyramid because I firmly believe that a healthy body and happy life start with a regular exercise plan and good eating habits. They are the two most critical parts of your battle against the aging process. Without them you won't have the strength and energy that you need to defend your body from disease and lead a full, productive life.

But don't underestimate the importance of the top of the pyramid, either. Good health and longevity are dependent on doing breast self-exams and getting mammograms, seeing a doctor regularly, and even flossing your teeth. And a positive attitude has been shown to boost your immune system and help stave off illnesses like heart disease and cancer—in my mind, it's one of the most underrated health and beauty tips around!

Just remember: Every little change, no matter how small it seems to you, is a plus. And it will serve as a foundation for the next change. Over time, as your new behaviors become habits, you'll be able to bring them all together easily and effortlessly.

THE 28-DAY CHALLENGE

The goal of this book is to help you develop positive habits that will last a lifetime. Setting small, short-term goals like wearing sunscreen or eating more fruits and veggies is important because these serve as stepping stones to your ultimate, long-term goals—things like more energy, better health and a positive self-image. Your goals, both short- and long-term, are important signposts that will keep you motivated and moving forward.

The Gauge Your Age quiz on pages 14 to 23 will help you determine what these personal goals are going to be. Of course, it's possible that you already know what you want to achieve, whether it's losing five pounds, eating to fight disease or regaining the radiance of your 20s. Either way, be sure to put it all down on paper.

At the end of each section of this book you'll find a place to write down your specific goals for the next four weeks. Lists can help you determine your priorities and stay focused on your mission. You can post your lists around the house, in your car or in your office. Carry copies in your pocketbook. The more reminders, the better—and not because I think that you're going to have a menopausal memory lapse!

Instead of just focusing on exercise or healthy eating goals, you'll work on mastering *one* goal from each of the five sections (exercise, diet, health, beauty and attitude) each week. That's a total of *five* weekly goals. I've designed it this way so that you grow to understand the importance and interrelatedness of all five parts of my Anti-Aging Pyramid and begin cultivating a balanced approach to staying young.

Because exercise is fundamental and everyone needs it, I've listed your goals for you. This is the minimum that I want you to do for good health and to get started down the road to a more youthful appearance. If you want to do more, feel free to scribble in your revised agenda for the weeks ahead. Your goals in other areas are, of course, up to you.

I know that some of you will be in a rush to completely overhaul your life and see those amazing age-defying results. But trying to make too many changes all at once can backfire. Instead we'll be tackling five goals at a time—one from each section of the pyramid per week. At the end of four weeks you'll review your progress and count how many successful changes you were able to make. Were you able to stick with your exercise goals? Have you been taking precautions against skin cancer? Are your eating habits improving or have you reverted back to living on junk food? If you don't achieve all your goals, don't despair. I don't expect you to get it all right the first time. Depending on how you fare in the first four weeks, you can continue working toward the same goals or set new ones.

Can you do it? Absolutely—if you're smart and committed and take it one step at a time. That's your 28-day challenge! To help ensure your success over the next four weeks, follow these five great tips:

1. Plan ahead. Break your weekly goals down into daily tasks, then get a day planner and write it all down. Schedule time for workouts, grocery shopping, skin care and other important routines. Be as specific as possible. At the outset of the first week make a detailed shopping list of items that you'll need to start your program—for instance, new workout shoes, a set of dumbbells, water bottles, sunscreen and a supply of healthy food. It's important to start off on the right foot, and the time you put into organizing and planning will pay off later.

2. Prevent pitfalls. If you've been on a variety of different weight loss diets—all of which have failed—or have never been able to stick with an exercise program, stop and think about what went wrong. (Indeed, about 95 percent of all dieters regain lost weight within a few years.) What can you learn from those experiences and how can you keep them from happening again? Knowing your specific barriers to success can help you overcome them. For instance, if last-minute meetings have kept you from getting to the gym after work, you may need to start working out in the morning. Or if you can't seem to resist your husband's chocolate ice cream, why not buy a lower-calorie alternative like frozen yogurt or fat-free pops to store in your freezer? The best offense is always a good defense!

3. Don't get discouraged. What if you blow it by bingeing on greasy pizza or downing a sinful piece of Death by Chocolate? What if your kids are sick and you miss two, three, four days of exercise in a row? Get right back on that horse and whatever happens, DON'T CALL IT QUITS! Remember, you're developing lifelong habits that will help you for years to come—and slowing down and reversing the aging process takes time. So a little slip here or there isn't going to topple your efforts if you resume your diet or exercise regimen the very next day. Furthermore, the ability to overcome adversity and bounce back is one of the greatest measures of success in life. So follow every little step back with a giant step forward.

4. Pat yourself on the back. Most of us spend way too much time being critical of ourselves: "I can't do this," "If only I was more of that." Instead of focusing on the negatives, why not accentuate the positives? You only lost three pounds? You also gained strength and muscle tone—and you're three pounds closer to your ultimate goal. To teach yourself to focus on the positives, give yourself a reward—a massage, a manicure, a shopping spree or a night out with friends—whenever you reach a goal. Or if you're on a budget, treat yourself to a bubble bath or an hour of reading magazines. Rewards will help keep you motivated to keep moving forward.

5. Update your goals. At the end of four weeks I want you to assess where you are and where you'd like to go next. Congratulate yourself for all the goals you were able to achieve. Renew your vows to master those you haven't. Think about what other improvements you'd like to make, set your goals and form a new plan for success.

Above all, be patient! You're creating a healthier lifestyle for yourself that will offer benefits both now and for the future. Change is good, but change takes time. If you find your enthusiasm waning, picture yourself slipping into those great jeans you had five years ago (a size smaller than the ones you're in now) or wearing a silky-smooth complexion. Stay committed and your efforts will pay off, I promise.

One last reminder: We're all unique, and what works for me may not exactly work for you. For example, I like to work out in the morning—it wakes me up, puts me in a good mood and gives me energy to greet the day (plus I get it over with!). Maybe you prefer going for a power walk at lunch or riding a stationary bike during the evening news. No problem! Simply use the information in this book to create your own personalized anti-aging plan.

Above all, take heart. We are a generation of smart, accomplished women. We all went through the 1960s, with Twiggy as the ideal female. But this is not about thinness—it's about wellness and it's about time.

2

The Gauge Your Age Quiz

Are you growing old gracefully? Or is your body already older than its years? How you look on the outside isn't always an accurate reflection of what's going on in the inside—and neither is the number of candles on your last birthday cake. To help you assess how your body is really aging, take the quiz on the following pages.

Like the book, my Gauge Your Age quiz is divided into five sections—exercise, nutrition, health, beauty and attitude. Answer all of the questions in each section, then tally up your score. Based on your results, you may want to spend a little more time focusing on certain sections of this book. For example, you may discover that your skin care routine is super but your eating habits need help. In that case, you'll want to make nutrition the focus of your personal anti-aging program.

Ready to put your lifestyle under the anti-aging microscope? Grab a pen or pencil and let's get started!

EXERCISE
1. How often do you take the stairs instead of the elevator?
   a. Never
   b. Rarely
   c. Occasionally
   d. As often as possible

2. How many hours of household activity (cleaning, yardwork, laundry, etc.) do you do each week?

   a. None
   b. 1 to 6 hours
   c. 6 to 12 hours
   d. Too much to count

3. How often do you exercise aerobically (walking, riding a
    stationary bike, playing tennis, etc.) for at least 30 minutes?
    a. Never
    b. 1 or 2 times per month
    c. 1 to 2 times per week
    d. 3 or more times per week

4. How long does it take you to walk one mile?
    a. More than 25 minutes
    b. 21 to 25 minutes
    c. 15 to 20 minutes
    d. Less than 15 minutes

5. When's the last time you lifted weights?
    a. More than 6 months ago
    b. 3 to 6 months ago
    c. A week ago
    d. Yesterday

6. How would you spend your ideal weekend?
    a. On the couch—I'm always exhausted
    b. Getting together with friends for dinner or a movie
    c. Gardening, cooking
    d. Staying active: long walks, playing tennis or going for a bike
        ride

7. How often do you stretch or do yoga?
    a. Never
    b. Once a month
    c. Once a week
    d. Every day

8. How long can you stand on one foot without losing your balance?
    a. Less than 5 seconds
    b. 5 to 10 seconds
    c. 10 to 30 seconds
    d. 30 to 60 seconds or longer

9. How often do you do abdominal exercises?
    a. Never
    b. Once a month
    c. Once a week
    d. Three to four days a week

Scoring:
Count your number of As, Bs, Cs and Ds.

What Your Score Means:
If you scored mostly As: A stands for ATROPHY—you need more ACTIVITY!
If you scored mostly Bs: BETTER but still a BUNCH of work to do.
If you scored mostly Cs: You're ready for a CHALLENGE—can you CLICK IT UP A NOTCH?
If you scored mostly Ds: You are a DOER. DON'T go DOWNHILL!

NUTRITION

1. What's your typical breakfast?
    a. Oatmeal with skim milk and a banana
    b. A bagel with cream cheese
    c. A latte and a muffin
    d. Nothing—you skip breakfast

2. What kind of supplements do you take?
    a. A daily multivitamin and a calcium supplement
    b. A daily multivitamin only
    c. Vitamin C when you feel a cold coming on
    d. None of the above

3. How much water do you drink daily?
    a. More than 8 glasses
    b. 4 glasses
    c. 1 or 2, if you can remember
    d. None

4. What's your typical lunch?
    a. A grilled chicken salad with vinaigrette dressing
    b. Tuna fish sandwich, chips and a Coke
    c. Cheeseburger, french fries, milkshake
    d. I skip lunch, then usually hit the vending machines by 4 P.M.

5. How many servings of fruits and vegetables do you eat on an average day?
   a. 5 to 8
   b. 3 to 5
   c. 1 to 2
   d. Does an orange soda count as fruit?

6. What are you most likely to reach for as a snack?
   a. A piece of fruit
   b. Baked chips and salsa
   c. Cheese, crackers, nuts
   d. A Snickers bar

7. How often do you eat soy products (tofu, soy milk, soy nuts, etc.)?
   a. Every day
   b. Occasionally
   c. Rarely
   d. What's soy?

8. What kind of milk do you drink?
   a. Nonfat or skim
   b. 1 or 2 percent
   c. Whole
   d. I don't drink milk

9. How often do you skip a meal?
   a. Never
   b. Maybe once or twice a month
   c. About once a week
   d. About once a day

10. What kind of breakfast cereal do you typically eat?
    a. Bran flakes
    b. Rice Krispies
    c. Cap'n Crunch
    d. Granola (not low-fat)

11. What type of beverage do you typically drink with meals?
    a. Water or herbal tea
    b. Juice
    c. Diet soda
    d. Alcohol, regular soda

12. How often do you feel "stuffed" from overeating?
    a. Almost never
    b. On weekends and holidays
    c. Once a week
    d. At every meal

Scoring:
Count your number of As, Bs, Cs and Ds.

What Your Score Means:
If you scored mostly As: You get APPLAUSE and a nutritional A-PLUS!
If you scored mostly Bs: Your eating habits aren't too BAD but could be BETTER.
If you scored mostly Cs: CAUTION! You need to make CHANGES that include CUTTING CALORIES and reducing your fat intake.
If you scored mostly Ds: DON'T wait a DAY to DITCH your DIET!

HEALTH

1. How would you rate your family health history?
    a. Excellent
    b. Good
    c. Fair, with some heart disease and cancer
    d. Poor or not sure

2. How much do you weigh?
    a. My weight is about right for my height
    b. I'm less than 15 pounds overweight
    c. I'm 15 to 30 pounds overweight
    d. I'm more than 30 pounds overweight

3. How often do you do breast self-exams?
    a. Once a month
    b. Twice a year
    c. Once a year
    d. Never

4. If you're over 40 or have a family history of breast cancer, how often do you get mammograms?
    a. Once a year
    b. Every year or two
    c. Every three years
    d. Never

5. How often do you see your gynecologist for a Pap smear?
   a. At least once a year
   b. Every other year
   c. Whenever I remember
   d. Never

6. How long ago did you quit smoking?
   a. I've never smoked
   b. More than 10 years ago
   c. Five to 10 years ago
   d. Less than 5 years ago

7. How often do you get a full dental exam?
   a. At least once a year
   b. Every other year
   c. Whenever I remember
   d. Never—I hate the dentist!

8. What does your daily oral hygiene routine involve?
   a. Brushing and flossing
   b. Brushing only
   c. Flossing only
   d. Neither

9. How often do you wear a seatbelt?
   a. Every time I get in a car
   b. Whenever I'm in the front seat of a car
   c. Whenever I remember
   d. Never

10. How often do you have your eyes examined?
    a. Once a year
    b. Every other year
    c. Whenever I have a problem
    d. I've never had my eyes examined

11. How often do you get screened for skin cancer?
    a. Once a year
    b. Every other year
    c. About every five years
    d. I've never been screened for skin cancer

12. What did your last colorectal screening show?
    a. No problems
    b. Polyps
    c. Blood in my stool
    d. Aren't colorectal screenings just for men?

13. What is your blood pressure?
    a. Normal
    b. Low
    c. High
    d. Who knows?

14. What is your total cholesterol?
    a. Under 200
    b. Between 200 and 240
    c. Above 240
    d. Don't know

Scoring:
Count your number of As, Bs, Cs and Ds.

What Your Score Means:
If you scored mostly As: You're ALERT and ACTIVE. A-OKAY!
If you scored mostly Bs: A BIT more effort will BUILD a BETTER BODY.
If you scored mostly Cs: Serious CHANGES are needed if you want to improve your health.
If you scored mostly Ds: DECIDE today to DO a 180-DEGREE change in lifestyle.

BEAUTY
1. What do you cleanse your face with?
    a. Soap and hot water
    b. Gentle cleanser made for my skin type and warm water
    c. Whatever's lying around
    d. I never wash my face

2. When do you apply moisturizer?
    a. I never wear moisturizer
    b. Every time I wash my face
    c. Once a day after my shower
    d. In the winter only

3. How often do you get or give yourself a facial?
   a. Never
   b. Every six weeks
   c. Once a year
   d. Never

4. How often do you use wrinkle-fighters like creams with alpha hydroxy acids or products containing Retinol?
   a. Never
   b. Several times a week
   c. Once a month
   d. Once every six months

5. How frequently do you shampoo your hair?
   a. Every day
   b. Every other day
   c. Once a week
   d. Whenever it looks dirty

6. How often do you use a hair conditioner?
   a. Never
   b. Every time I wash my hair
   c. A couple of times a week
   d. Whenever I remember

7. On average, how much do you sleep?
   a. Less than six hours per night
   b. 8 or more hours per night
   c. Between 7 and 8 hours per night
   d. Between 6 and 7 hours per night

8. When you're going to be out in the sun, what do you wear for sun protection?
   a. Nothing—I like getting a little healthy color
   b. Sunscreen on all exposed areas, a hat, protective clothing and sunglasses
   c. Sunscreen on all exposed areas
   d. Sunscreen on my face only

9. How often do you do facial exercises?
   a. Never
   b. At least twice a week

    c. Maybe once a month
    d. Once in a blue moon

Scoring:
Count your number of As, Bs, Cs and Ds.

What Your Score Means:
If you scored mostly As: ALERT! Your APPEARANCE will suffer if you don't ATTEND to it ASAP.
If you scored mostly Bs: BRAVO—you're doing your BEST to preserve your gorgeous BEAUTY.
If you scored mostly Cs: You're CLOSE but your CHOICES still COULD be better.
If you scored mostly Ds: You're not completely in the DARK, but you could be DOING much more.

ATTITUDE

1. You're driving on a freeway when someone cuts you off. You
    a. Honk furiously and tailgate the offender
    b. Break down into tears and imagine the awful accident that almost happened
    c. Get off at the next exit and take a longer route
    d. Wave and keep driving—it's only traffic

2. You ask a salesperson for help finding a size 12, and she says, "Go look in the racks." You
    a. Demand to see her supervisor
    b. Wonder why this always happens to you
    c. Walk out
    d. Reply, "Why didn't I think of that?" and help yourself

3. When you try on bathing suits, you
    a. Complain about the bad lighting and leave in a huff
    b. Suck in your tummy—every year it seems to get worse
    c. Head straight for the one-piece with the long skirt
    d. Reach for the bright blue suit (it's your color!) and reaffirm your vow to exercise more

4. When a friend asks you to go hiking, you say
    a. No way—I hate hiking
    b. Oh, no, you're much better at it—I'd hold you back
    c. Let's try a less challenging walk
    d. Sounds like an adventure—let's go!

5. Your friend gives you a container of bath salts for your birthday. You think
    a. She'd know by now that I only take showers
    b. We never exchange gifts—and I didn't get anything for her birthday
    c. I'll keep it and give it to someone else
    d. What a thoughtful present—I can't wait to use it

6. You have a spat with a close friend. You
    a. Call mutual friends and gossip about her
    b. Spend days stewing about it—and consume a chocolate cake
    c. Decide to avoid her for a while
    d. Call her immediately, apologize and suggest lunch

7. Somebody makes a comment about your weight. You
    a. Tell him or her to buzz off
    b. Hide in a bathroom and cry, then get mad at yourself for being so fat
    c. Justify it by flipping through magazines for larger women
    d. Use it as the inspiration you needed to start working out and eating right

8. You've have a rotten day at work. You
    a. Swear that you hate your boss and throw the phone out the window
    b. Wish that you could leave your job but are convinced you wouldn't get a better one
    c. Go home, watch mindless TV and block it out
    d. Call a close friend and brainstorm about what you can do to improve the situation

Scoring:
Count your number of As, Bs, Cs and Ds.

What Your Score Means:
If you scored mostly As: You're ANGRY—which only ADDS to your problems.
If you scored mostly Bs: Your BAD self-image is holding you BACK from making BENEFICIAL changes.
If you scored mostly Cs: Instead of CHOOSING a CHALLENGE, you opt for the COMFORTABLE—which gets you nowhere.
If you scored mostly Ds: DELIGHTFUL! You focus on the positive and DON'T let little things get you DOWN.

The Gauge Your Age Quiz

If you didn't do as well on the Gauge Your Age quiz as you'd hoped, don't get discouraged. This is just the first step toward a brand-new, healthier you—and you've learned something valuable already. Remember: Knowledge is power when it comes to staying fit and protecting yourself against disease. So it's time to make use of this new knowledge and take action!

By starting today, you CAN change your future and turn back the clock. Are you ready to find out what it takes to build and maintain a strong, balanced, beautiful body—both inside and out? We'll be talking about exercise first, the base of my pyramid. So take a deep breath and flex those muscles as you turn the page and get started.

3

Exercise: Burn Back the Clock!

Last summer, I spent several weeks filming my television show on the beautiful island of Maui. The very first day, out of the corner of my eye, I noticed an attractive woman watching me. She came every morning after that. On the last day of filming, I was so curious that I went over and introduced myself and said I couldn't help but notice that she walked on the beach every day and always stopped to watch my film crew. She was delighted and said she had been a fan for years and had been doing my video "Hips, Thighs and Buttocks." My jaw dropped when she told me she was turning 60!

When I began to write this book, I asked the woman, Bernita Dawson, to share her success story:

Dear Denise,

I discovered your videos twelve years ago. You said if I did the video every day, it would make a difference, and you were right! I was in pretty good shape at the time but needed to firm up, so I gave it a try. It really does work, and I've been at it ever since. I've recommended the video to several friends and, in fact, just recently ordered another copy for a friend. Your daily advice, "strong body, strong mind," helped motivate me to go to college. . . . I was able to earn my bachelor's degree just three years ago and continue to take classes. It truly is a great way to keep the mind active, as well as being a wonderful experience. I am very proud of myself, and as you suggested, I am worth it.

Since turning 60 last year, I am plagued with more aches and pains, feelings of fatigue, dry skin and some insomnia. I find it harder to keep my weight down and keep in shape. But because of your influence, working out has become a way of life for me, and I'm better able to deal with these nuisances and keep my body fit. You are a prime example of what you can look like if you follow a fitness plan. You're a great motivator. . . . Thanks, Denise, you're terrific!

Bernita is a perfect example of how my pyramid works, and how it can help you turn back the clock. Exercise is the most important level—the foundation—of the program. Without physical activity, your body may age prematurely. Your bones may become brittle, putting you at risk of debilitating fractures. You're more likely to feel stiff when you get up out of a chair or to experience soreness in your hips and knees. New research shows that the majority of those aches and pains are actually the result of atrophy, not old age.

Furthermore, exercise is, without a doubt, the most effective way to battle those extra pounds that sneak up on us as we get older. Countless women have told me that they've tried a thousand diets and nothing seems to work. But there's a simple reason that most diets fail, and it's because dieting destroys your metabolism—period. And in order to lose weight, you need to kick your metabolism into high gear, not turn it off.

When you severely restrict your calories, your body goes into "starvation mode." Your resting metabolic rate (the rate at which your body burns calories for energy) will decrease, because your body thinks you are actually starving and wants to conserve energy. Therefore you stop burning calories efficiently. It also begins to "self-cannibalize," burning muscle instead of fat. If you really want to lose those love handles and keep your youthful shape, you need to jump-start your metabolism. The exercises in this book will help you do just that.

For any woman over 40, a pouchy tummy and flabby thighs aren't inevitable. Through strength training and aerobics you can build the muscle and burn the fat necessary to keep your metabolism revved up and reclaim your waistline.

With the right exercises, you can tone your hips, thighs, tummy and other areas that have started to sag. A droopy rear end and jiggly upper arms aren't your destiny—they're simply the signs of underdeveloped muscles!

In addition, researchers now know that regular exercise can help stave off heart disease, stroke, diabetes, osteoporosis and certain types of cancer. According to the American Heart Association, about 12 percent of deaths in the United States each year are blamed on lack of reg-

Remember: In order to remove one pound of fat from your body, you need to burn 3,500 calories.

ular physical activity. The association declared that weight lifting does in fact improve cardiovascular health. Strength training improves the body's ability to regulate insulin levels, reducing the odds of getting diabetes—a major risk factor for heart disease. It also reduces cholesterol, especially the "bad" LDL cholesterol. Even if you've been a sofa spud all of your life, starting a regular exercise program NOW can help you live longer, according to a study reported in the *American Heart Journal.* In the study the most physically active men and women were about 39 to 42 percent less likely to die than their counterparts who didn't exercise.

And the health benefits go beyond the heart. In a Harvard University study of women ages 40 to 65, the women who exercised the most had almost half the risk of stroke of those who exercised the least. The results held true even for those who did more moderate exercise, like brisk walking. Even subjects who had been sedentary but became active later in life experienced the benefits.

Sitting makes you stiff, sleepy and slow!

But best of all, being fit feels fantastic! (Thanks to those beta-endorphins—the body's natural pleasure chemicals—which kick in when you exercise.) And working out, as my friend Bernita found, does boost your self-esteem—the more skill and stamina you develop, the better you'll feel about yourself and all that life has to offer.

As you know, exercise has always been a key part of my life. I'm lucky that Jeff and I have space in our home for a treadmill, a mini-trampoline, a yoga mat, a stationary bike and sets of weights—it makes it easy to work out even on the most hectic days. My husband, who's turning 50, plays tennis and does weight training every day. Because I stay in shape, I feel better when I get dressed, and I don't want to hide under a big T-shirt when I hit the beach. My 43-year-old body feels ready for anything, including shooting hoops with Katie and Kelly, a

---

Denise's Top 6 Pep Talks

The long-term benefits of exercise are important, but let's not forget what it can do for you TODAY. Here are six mantras to carry with you and recite whenever you need a little inspiration.

- I always feel a deep sense of calm after exercising.

- It will help me stay fit.

- My clothes will fit better.

- I'll sleep better.

- My skin looks bright and rosy after a workout.

- Food tastes better because I've earned it.

game of tennis with my husband, a three-mile walk with a friend or doing flips off the diving board. I thank God every day that I have the strength and energy to work full time, take care of my husband and kids and be there for my family and friends.

Remember: Getting wider and slower and less able to do things isn't a fact of life. If you invest a little time and effort now, you can stop those changes from taking place—and reverse the ones that already have. Adopting a regular exercise program does take hard work and it won't always be fun, but your efforts will pay off—I guarantee it! You CAN turn back the hands of time—and the sooner you start, the better.

THE FOUR TYPES OF ANTI-AGING EXERCISE

Women over 40 need a balanced program designed to develop four fitness essentials: aerobic or cardiovascular conditioning, strength, flexibility and balance. What about those fabulous-looking women who *only* do aerobic workouts or *only* do yoga? Certainly doing one form of activity is better than doing nothing. But you'll do your body a favor if you have the time and energy to incorporate these four different types of exercise into your regular fitness program.

Aerobic Activity

"Burn Back the Clock"
"Blast Away Fat"

Aerobics refers to any exercise that gets your heart pumping, such as running, walking, biking, swimming or rowing. Your heart is a muscle that pumps blood through your body to carry oxygen to your cells and remove waste. Aerobic exercise strengthens the heart muscle and lowers blood pressure and cholesterol. This is good news for us, as the risk of heart disease rises sharply in postmenopausal women as a result of estrogen deficiency. Aerobic exercise, some studies suggest, can reduce your risk of heart disease by more than 40 percent.

Regular aerobic workouts are crucial for anyone who wants to live a long, healthy, active life, control weight, tone muscles and improve circulation. They give you energy and stamina for everyday life. The harder you get your heart pumping, the better—but I don't adhere to the "no pain, no gain" philosophy. Even light to moderate aerobic activities can help reduce blood pressure and fight the aging process.

Regular aerobic activity can also enhance digestion and bowel regularity, as well as regulate blood sugar. Aerobic activity increases your metabolic rate, so you can actually stop dieting and eat normally without gaining weight. Exercise increases muscle mass, and that increases your ability to burn calories.

In addition, aerobic exercise can alleviate symptoms of menopause. In one study of more than 1,600 women, sedentary women were twice as likely to report hot flashes as physically active women. Exercise also staves off bone loss. Women can lose up to 1 percent of total bone mass yearly from age 40 until menopause. During the first 5 to 10 years after menopause, annual bone loss averages about 2 percent—which means that by the time you are 60 you could lose nearly 30 percent of your bone mass!

In my Stop the Clock exercise program (I also like to call it "Burn Back the Clock"), you'll be doing 30 minutes of cardiovascular exercise three or four times a week. That's the *minimum* needed to protect your heart, burn fat and manage your weight. If 30 minutes of cardio sounds next to impossible, rest assured that you can work up to it. If you can't keep up with a workout in the beginning, slow down and do what you can. Moving counts, so just keep moving! The next time you exercise, you'll do a little more, and a little more, and then a little more—and pretty soon you won't remember when you couldn't do a full 30 minutes.

If you're a veteran exerciser, you may want to do more. Either way, don't overdo it, especially in the beginning. If you try to do too much too soon, you'll only end up tired and sore, which could soften your resolve to keep exercising.

Once you do work up to it, there may be days that you absolutely don't have time for a full 30-minute workout. My solution: Do what you can, even if it's just for 5 or 10 minutes. It may not seem worthwhile to change clothes and get sweaty for such a short time, but 5 or 10 minutes is still enough to burn a few calories and give your metabolism a tiny kick.

There are a variety of aerobic workouts that you can do to strengthen your cardiovascular system and burn calories. I've listed some of my favorites below. And remember: Aerobic activity doesn't always have to mean putting on workout clothes or huffing and puffing on a treadmill. In a pinch, it can include scrubbing your bathtub or a brisk walk to buy a bottle of water. Or put the stereo on and dance, dance, dance to a few of your favorite songs!

Even if it isn't a cardio day, you'll benefit by doing some form of aerobic activity, whether it's walking the dog, running up and down the stairs or taking a spin on the stationary bike (more about that on page 41). As you learn to incorporate exercise into your everyday life, some of these activities should become second nature. You won't feel like you're working out twice. You'll simply experience the exercise high and the joy of slipping into pants that are loose instead of tight!

The Best Cardio Workouts for Your Age Group

Below is a list of some of the best heart-healthy workouts for your age group. I'm certainly not suggesting that you limit yourself to these workouts. If you wanted to, you could do aqua aerobics in your 40s or, if you're in good enough shape, jog well into your 60s and 70s. It's all up to your ability and preferences. This is simply a guide to help lead you to activities that you can pursue safely and with optimal results as you grow older.

In Your 40s

Jogging and running	Race walking
Kickboxing	Aerobic dance
Power walking	Rope jumping
Cycling	Stair climbing
Elliptical machine	Rowing
Swimming	Hiking
Tennis	Cross-country skiing
Power yoga	

In Your 50s

Jogging	Power walking
Cycling	Stair climbing
Elliptical machine	Rowing machine
Low-impact aerobics	Swimming
Hiking	Tennis
Power yoga	

In Your 60s

Power walking	Elliptical machine
Aqua aerobics	Swimming
Cross-country skiing	Hiking
Tennis	Dancing
Power yoga	

Strength Training

Strong muscles are one of the best defenses against aging. Muscle burns three times more calories than fat does, so the more muscle you have, the more calories your body burns, even while you're sleeping. Besides boosting your metabolism, strong muscles can help protect your bones from osteoporosis and improve your posture. When muscles are toned and taut, nothing can droop or sag!

After 40 our muscles shrink at a rate of about 1 percent each year unless we do regular strength-training exercises. Aerobic exercise like walking or cross-country skiing can help strengthen your muscles, but not enough to compensate for the loss. The best way to prevent and reverse muscle loss is by strength training: weight-bearing exercises specifically designed to strengthen and build your muscles.

Luckily, it's never too late to rebuild muscle, and you don't need to pump iron like a body builder to benefit. New studies on strength training suggest it's never too late to start. In one study 10 nursing home residents from ages 86 to 96 enrolled in a program of weight-lifting exercises. Of those who completed the eight-week program, thigh muscle strength increased an average of 74 percent. More important, five of the formerly frail residents increased their gait speed by nearly 50 percent, and two of the subjects no longer needed canes to walk. Strengthening their muscles also helped to increase bone density and reduce their risk of debilitating fractures.

Evidence also suggests that weight training can lower resting blood pressure by 2–4 percent, decreasing the risk of heart disease and stroke. According to a recent study at Northern Illinois University, a regimen of single sets of 8 to 15 repetitions of several different exercises two or three times a week can make the difference.

There are several different ways to strength-train. You can lift hand weights or dumbbells, which you'll be doing in my Stop the Clock program. You can use weight machines at a gym. Or you can do exercises like push-ups or Pilates, which use your own body weight as resistance—another muscle-building technique that you'll be utilizing later in this book.

When I talk about lifting weights, many of you may picture the serious body builder we've all seen on television and think, "No way. I don't want to look like that!" But you needn't worry about bulking up like

Success Story

Sally had been active all her life, regularly playing tennis, taking brisk walks and occasionally riding her bike around the neighborhood. Then, at age 61, she discovered strength training. A new fitness club opened up in her area, and she decided to see what they had to offer. During her free introductory session, a personal trainer set her up with a weight-training program using machines in the gym. Seven years later, she has dropped from a size 14 to a size 12, firmed up her tummy and, at a recent reunion, was the only one of her high school friends who could wear a sleeveless shirt and still smile. "At first I was intimidated by the weight machines and doubted whether what I was doing would really make a difference," she says. But her gym has lots of over-60 members and makes an effort to be senior-friendly by offering special classes and follow-up workouts with trainers. "After trying the machines a few times, I figured out how to use them," she says. "And the results have been great. I not only look better, I play tennis better than I did 10 or 20 years ago."

Exercise: Burn Back the Clock!

Arnold Schwarzenegger: Most women don't have enough of the hormone testosterone to "get big." In fact, lifting weights will have the opposite effect. As you replace fat with muscle, you'll look and feel leaner. Your clothes will fit better, and your body will be tighter and firmer. More muscle = less fat. Research proves it!

Training for Flexibility and Balance

In your teens and 20s you could touch your toes, move from sitting to standing without a single crack or pop, and do a cheerleader split—no problem. But as you've hit middle age, you've no doubt started to notice changes. Your muscles feel stiff and tight when you wake up in the morning (arthritis, decreasing ability of your muscles and connective tissue to elongate) or sit for long periods of time. No longer can you touch your toes or jump up from the floor with ease—and attempting a split would be suicide!

Arthritis currently affects more than 40 million Americans and will affect 60 million by the year 2020. People with this often debilitating pain—caused by the breakdown of joint cartilage—limit their activities. Research shows that appropriate exercise is vital to managing arthritis symptoms. It increases flexibility and strength and reduces pain and fatigue. Stretching helps pump vital nutrients to your muscles and tendons, which helps keep them healthy and minimizes your risk of injury. It also stimulates the production of joint lubricants (synovial fluid) and helps prevents adhesions. As circulation increases, so does your energy. Your legs, back, neck and shoulders loosen up, relieving aches and stiffness. As your muscles lengthen, your posture improves and you look taller, thinner and leaner. You'll feel stronger and steadier in all your favorite activities; your golf swing will lengthen and you'll be able to make those difficult shots on the tennis court.

Balance also starts to deteriorate in your 40s as your muscles weaken and your nerve receptors lose sensitivity. You may not notice the occasional stumbles or wobbling at first, but over time those little changes become more and more apparent. Your tennis game declines and sports like skiing become more difficult. You become nervous walking on uneven terrain and dread climbing up a flight of stairs at a basketball arena. Overall, you start to slow down and limit your activities, all in an effort to avoid falling.

The good news is, you *can* improve your balance and minimize that wobbly feeling by strengthening your muscles, especially the stabilizing muscles in your core (abdominals and lower back) and on both sides of your ankles. A Wake Forest University study found that aerobics or weight training can improve balance in adults with this condition, as well as reduce knee pain. As you'll see in my workout on page 70, balance exercises aren't difficult or time-consuming—and they can help you regain your steady footing and your confidence to take up hiking, chase your kids and grandkids around the yard and enjoy all that life has to offer.

MAKING TIME FOR EXERCISE

When you're young, your body seems to take care of itself. You can eat whatever you want without gaining weight. You have an endless supply of energy. Your blood pressure and your cholesterol are on target. You feel great. Then, gradually, things start to change. Your weight creeps up, your joints get achy, your blood pressure rises, and your cholesterol level goes through the roof. All of a sudden, you have real problems—blocked arteries, an underactive thyroid, severe arthritis, maybe even depression.

With a regular exercise program, it all could have been prevented.

I know that you're busy. Maybe you have a full- or part-time job, a family to feed, a house to clean, aging parents to look after, and countless meetings. You do it all. But you also know that you're overweight and out of shape and that you should do something about it.

It's easy to make excuses. At times there are going to be things that seem more important than getting in a workout. But nothing is more important than your health—not work, not cleaning the bathroom, not surfing the Internet and certainly not that juicy TV movie. The longer you wait to get started, the harder it will get—and the bigger your problems are going to be.

Even with the busiest schedule, it's possible to find time for exercise. I'm living proof! How do over-40 women like me find time for exercise when we're juggling a million things? We don't. We MAKE time. In other words, we carve time out of our hectic schedules because we know the importance of staying in shape and the consequences of not doing it.

Bottom line: You need to make exercise a top priority. How? Start by sitting down and making a list of all your exercise obstacles and what you can do to overcome them. If long hours on the job keep you from exercising, bring exercise to work. Lace up your sneakers and walk up the stairs or around the block during your 10-minute coffee break. If you're open-minded and creative enough, every exercise obstacle will have a solution. Researchers at the University of Arkansas recently found that in women over 50 everyday weight-bearing activities like yard work (pruning a hedge or planting vegetables) can build bone mass and may help prevent osteoporosis.

I'm the first one to admit that exercise can be a drag. There are lots of mornings that I'd rather curl up and watch the *Today* show than lace up my shoes and go for a run. But I do it anyway because I know how important it is and how much better I'll feel afterward. Besides offering countless health benefits, exercise puts me in a good mood, gives me clarity and allows me to *really* enjoy my food throughout the rest of the day.

If you're starting a fitness program for the first time, you may find it difficult or uncomfortable at first. Rest assured that your workouts will get easier. As you get stronger and build endurance, working out will become less uncomfortable, and if you play your cards right, you will begin to enjoy it. Your body generally wants whatever it's given. If you sit, it will want to sit. If you move, it will want to keep moving.

On those days that you'd rather get a tooth drilled than exercise, promise yourself that you'll do five minutes' worth—even if it's just a power walk around the block or walking up and down the stairs for five minutes. It's amazing how many times those five minutes turn into more. Even a small amount of activity can burn calories and leave you feeling energized!

If you think you're being selfish by taking time out from your other obligations and activities for a workout, consider the oxygen mask analogy. When we travel by plane, we're always instructed to put on our own oxygen mask before helping family members in the case of an emergency. The same is true for exercise and a healthy lifestyle. If you don't take care of yourself, you may not be able to care for your loved ones. This isn't a doomsday scenario. Instead it's a strong reminder that any effort to preserve your health benefits your family, too. If you feel well, you'll be more pleasant to spend time with. You'll have more energy for trips to the amusement park or cheering your little slugger on at his or her baseball game. Most important, you'll be more likely to be around for them in the years to come.

> **Research shows that sedentary people can increase their life spans by up to three years simply by moving more throughout the day.**

FIDGETCIZE!™

Many people assume that I'm an exercise fanatic, working out for hours each day. In fact, I do only 30 minutes of "official" exercise daily. But I never miss an opportunity to move, even when I'm stuck in an elevator or brushing my teeth. I call it Fidgetcize, and I really rely on these little extras to keep me fit and feeling my best, especially when I'm on the road for work or under a lot of stress.

While a structured program designed to build aerobic conditioning, strength, flexibility and balance is your best anti-aging insurance policy, you can fight flab and improve your health just by being more active in your daily life. Research shows that simple habits like taking the stairs instead of an escalator can keep your body limber and lean. Even small movements like tapping your toes may help you maintain a youthful figure. According to a study conducted at the Mayo Clinic in Rochester, Minnesota, people who fidget—you know, high-energy, restless types who can't sit still—burn more calories than natural-born couch potatoes. Plus, you can burn up to 500 calories each day if you fidget! So start Fidgetcizing.

There are other benefits besides burning calories, of course: Every time you push a vacuum around the house or simply get up from a chair and stretch, you send blood coursing through your body. That blood delivers vital nutrients to your muscles and joints to help keep them healthy. It also can give you an instant energy boost! Increased circulation can combat sluggishness and make you more mentally alert, whether you're sitting in traffic or an important business meeting.

Make it your goal to get up once every hour and move for one to two minutes. Go for a short walk, march in place, climb up and down a flight of stairs. Do standing leg lifts or mini-squats while you wash dishes or brush your teeth. If you're trapped in a car or on an airplane, try "invisible" exercises like tummy tucks or butt squeezes. It may seem silly, but if it works, who cares? You'll be laughing your way to the size 10 rack.

The hardest part about Fidgetcizing is getting in the habit. I've trained myself to keep moving, and so can you. One way to do it is to post little reminders to yourself around the house or in your office. Or try to get the rest of your family and your friends on the Fidgetcize program. Turn it into a game—she who fidgets most wins! Whether you're doing arm curls with grocery bags or tapping your toes on the train, you'll be burning extra calories, building stronger muscles and keeping your body energized.

Start right now by tapping your toes as you continue to read or putting down the book and stretching your muscles: Extend your arms overhead as high as possible, then lower your arms and do shoulder

Remember: Exercise anywhere—anytime. Your muscles don't know if you're in the kitchen or a fancy gym.

Easy Ways to Fidgetcize

I love turning listless moments into exercise opportunities. Here are some of my favorite techniques for fidgeting my way to a better body:

- Squeezing my gluteal (buttocks) muscles for 10 seconds and releasing while brushing my teeth

- Working my calf muscles by standing on tiptoe, then lowering and rising, while standing at the copy machine

- Doing overhead stretches while waiting at a stoplight

rolls, waist twists (turn your body to the right, then twist it to the left) and calf raises (lift your heels up and down). I bet you feel better already. Not a bad way to burn hundreds of extra calories a day, wouldn't you say?

THE STOP THE CLOCK WORKOUT PLAN

Aerobic workouts, strength training, flexibility and balance exercises—it sounds like a lot to learn and remember, right? To help, I've created a comprehensive program designed to help you tackle all four anti-aging essentials. Just think of all that can be attained in less than an hour each day: a strong heart and healthy lungs; muscles that look strong and lean, with no jiggly-wiggly; and a trim, nimble body for scrambling after a toddler or up a mountain trail without fear of falling. Best of all, you'll feel better inside—younger, happier, livelier!

In the Stop the Clock plan, you'll be doing the minimum amount of exercise necessary for good health and to slow the aging process.

WEEKLY SCHEDULE
Cardio: 30 minutes, 3 to 4 times per week
Strength Training: 30 minutes, 2 to 3 times per week
Flexibility/Balance Exercises: 5 to 10 minutes, 6 times per week
Anti-Gravity Exercises: 10 minutes, 2 or 3 times per week (optional)
Extra Bonus Exercises: Just pick your "area" of concern

Any exercise that you do above and beyond this basic prescription will Stop the Clock, or *reverse* the aging process. Now, before you start groaning, let me remind you that exercise doesn't have to mean putting on workout clothes and getting sweaty. In other words, add a few extra tummy tucks on the train, a short walk before dinner and a couple of yoga poses during *Jeopardy,* and you'll be turning back the clock. It's that easy!

In this section, you'll find a weight-loss Walking Workout as well as specific routines designed to increase strength, flexibility and balance. I've also provided gravity-defying toning exercises to help you target and tone your specific trouble spots—you know, places like your thighs and the backs of your arms that may have started to sag and cause "mirror" anxiety. These moves are optional, but I recommend giving them a try. Nothing makes you look and feel years younger than firm thighs in shorts or toned arms in a sleeveless top.

In the following weeks I also want you to get in the habit of moving more throughout your day. While your daily workouts will help stop the clock, Fidgetcize is the key to "turning back the clock." Yes, you can whittle your waistline and increase your longevity just by being more active in your daily life. Each time you get up from your chair and move, you're burning calories and fighting middle-age spread. Every little move you make, no matter how small, is a plus. So stand up right now and stretch. You'll be glad you did!

If you're like many of my Lifetime-TV viewers, "lack of time" is your biggest obstacle to maintaining a regular workout regimen. So I've designed a program that makes it easier to fit it in. While you should aim to do 30 minutes of continuous activity during your aerobic workouts, your strength workouts can be split up—10 minutes in the morning and 10 minutes before dinner. I've made it easy for you by creating 10-minute routines for you to mix and match.

At the end of this chapter you'll find a Progress Report and a Workout Log. The Progress Report includes five, simple fitness tests. Take these quick tests at the start of the Stop the Clock program, then repeat the tests again at the end of four weeks. Record your results in the space provided—and be sure to give yourself a pat on the back for all your successes. In the Workout Log you'll find space to jot down the date and duration of each exercise session as well as how you felt afterward. Keeping a written record of your workouts is a great way to keep yourself honest and motivated.

Don't worry if you do miss a workout or two during the course of a week; don't get discouraged. You haven't blown it, so don't even think about "throwing in" the towel. Successful people don't quit in the face of adversity—they get determined. So pick right back up where you left off.

For the next four weeks I'm going to be your very own personal trainer and coach. Feel as though I am with you each day. Scientists believe it takes three to four weeks to form a new habit, so really give it your all for these next 28 days. Your goal is to make exercise as much a part of your lifestyle as brushing your teeth. So I personally believe that you can make working out such a part of your mind-set and daily routine that you just won't want to quit. You can do it—believe in yourself, and it will be so!

Getting Started

Fitness after 40 is no different from fitness at 20, depending on what you've been doing with yourself. If you've never exercised before, you're overweight, you're a smoker, you're over age 60 or you have a chronic health condition (cardiovascular disease, high blood pressure, osteoporosis, kidney disease, liver disease or arthritis), consult your physician before getting started. Otherwise, follow these five basic rules for the road:

Start slowly. If you've never exercised before or it's been three months or more since your last workout, you'll need to ease into your new exercise program. Even die-hard aerobic exercisers who haven't worked out in a while due to illness or other reasons don't automatically pick up where they left off. They start gradually. Beginners should start by doing about 10 minutes a day five times a week. During Week 2 increase your time to 20 minutes. By the third week you should be up to 30 minutes per workout—the minimum amount needed to Stop the Clock.

Always warm up. Before doing any type of exercise, even if it's just a round of golf, I recommend doing a quick warm-up (about three to five minutes) to get your muscles ready for action. Any light activity such as walking or marching in place will increase the flow of blood and oxygen to your muscles, preparing them for the stress to come. Once your muscles are warm, lightly stretch the ones that you plan to use during your workout. This will help loosen up your muscles, so you're less likely to strain yourself or develop injuries.

Dress appropriately. Proper clothing and footwear is crucial for both comfort and safety reasons. Lycra workout wear or any loose, stretchy outfit will do. Try to avoid cotton, as it tends to get wet and heavy when you perspire. Ideally, you should wear shoes that are specifically designed for the activity you'll be doing. A sturdy pair of cross-trainers will work for most activities. If you plan to make walking your primary form of aerobic activity, consider investing in a pair of walking shoes. Here are some tips for buying shoes:

- Have your feet measured while standing.
- Try on both shoes and walk around.
- Buy for the larger foot.
- Shop for shoes in the afternoon, when feet tend to swell.
- Select shoes with good flexibility at the ball of the foot.
- Replace after six months, depending on wear.

Most important, your feet should feel comfy (with enough wiggle room around the toes) and have plenty of cushioning and support to help absorb any pounding to the joints. Also, if you're prone to shin-splints, make sure your shoe has a good arch support since shin-splints can result from a fallen arch or flat feet.

Hydrate, hydrate, hydrate. While the average person should drink 8 to 10 glasses of water a day (we'll learn more about water in the nutrition section), your body will need even more to replace excess water lost during exercise. Aim to drink a big glass of water before and after each exercise session—or keep a bottle of water nearby and sip, sip, sip throughout your workout. It will help boost your energy and keep your muscles at peak performance.

Breathe! Breathing is our energizing life force. Each breath fills our bodies with oxygen. Oxygen supplies necessary nutrients to every cell, giving us the energy to keep moving. Deep breathing can help us lengthen and stretch a muscle just a little bit further or walk another half mile. (You'll find details on breathing in the various workouts.) Breathing is essential to any exercise that we do. It's also an easy, terrific way to energize your body or tackle a stressful moment (more about that later on in the book).

Tips for Getting Started

- Check with your doctor first if you've never exercised before, you have health problems or you're over 60.
- Start slowly—work for at least 10 minutes; aim for 30.
- Always warm up.
- Wear appropriate clothing and shoes.
- Drink plenty of water.
- Watch your breathing.

Planning Your Workouts

Because we are all so busy it's so important to schedule your workouts. Setting aside a specific time for each exercise session makes you more likely to follow through with it. So before starting, take out a calendar and map out your workouts for the next four weeks. Don't forget that your strength and flexibility/balance workouts can be split up and spread throughout your day. For example, you can do half of your 30-minute strength workout in the morning and half in the evening while you watch TV. For aerobic workouts, you should aim for a full 30 minutes of continuous activity—but when your schedule won't permit it, you can divide them up, too.

To give you an idea of all your different scheduling options, I've designed four sample weekly workout plans (page 40). All four weekly plans include four days of cardio and three days of strength training. If you're really crunched for time, be sure to do a minimum of three cardio and two strength-training workouts per week. I've included the optimal length of each workout as well, although many of you will need to work up to those levels. Don't forget to skip a day between strength-training workouts—your muscles need 48 hours to recover. And remember that these are just ideas—only you know how to best schedule exercise into your busy days.

DAILY DOER PLAN

Monday   cardio (total: 30 min.)
Tuesday   strength PLUS flexibility/balance (total: 30–40 min.)
Wednesday   cardio (total: 30 min.)
Thursday   strength PLUS flexibility/balance (total: 30–40 min.)
Friday   cardio (total: 30 min.)
Saturday   strength PLUS flexibility/balance (total: 30–40 min.)
Sunday   cardio (total: 30 min.)

TIME-CRUNCH 4-DAY PLAN

Monday   cardio PLUS strength PLUS flexibility/balance
              (total: 60–70 min.)
Tuesday   OFF
Wednesday   cardio PLUS strength PLUS flexibility/balance
              (total: 60–70 min.)
Thursday   OFF
Friday   cardio PLUS strength PLUS flexibility/balance
              (total: 60–70 min.)
Saturday   cardio (total: 30 min.)
Sunday   OFF

WEEKEND FREE PLAN

Monday   cardio PLUS strength PLUS flexibility/balance
              (total: 60–70 minutes)
Tuesday   cardio (total: 30 minutes)
Wednesday   strength PLUS flexibility/balance (total: 30–40
              minutes)
Thursday   cardio (total: 30 minutes)
Friday   cardio PLUS strength PLUS flexibility/balance
              (total: 60–70 minutes)
Saturday   OFF
Sunday   OFF

WEEKEND FAT BLASTER PLAN

Monday   strength PLUS flexibility/balance (total: 30–40
              minutes)
Tuesday   cardio (total: 30 minutes)

Wednesday	cardio PLUS strength PLUS flexibility/balance (total: 60–70 minutes)
Thursday	OFF
Friday	strength PLUS flexibility/balance (total: 30–40 minutes)
Saturday	cardio (total : 30 minutes)
Sunday	cardio (total: 30 minutes)

MY WALKING WORKOUT

One of our biggest obstacles to regular exercise is time—our busy schedules always seem to get in the way. That's just one of the reasons why I included this Walking Workout in my book. Walking is a heart-healthy workout that you can really tailor to your schedule. All you need is a good pair of shoes and socks, so you can walk your way to better health and a slimmer body practically anytime, anywhere! I love to walk—it's such a great way to work out!

No matter what your age or physical condition, walking is an ideal way to maintain your youthful shape. To lose one pound of body fat, you need to burn approximately 3,500 calories. When you walk at a brisk pace, you burn about four calories per minute—or about 120 calories in half an hour. Go for a brisk 30-minute walk every day and you'll burn about 43,800 calories in a year. If your eating habits remain the same, you'll drop about 12.5 pounds in 12 months. Cut your calories, too, and you'll lose even more.

How Many Calories Can You Burn in 30 Minutes?

If you walk slowly (2.0 to 2.5 mph) on a flat surface
You'll burn about 90 calories (3 calories/minute)

If you walk at a slow to moderate pace (3.0 mph) on a flat surface
You'll burn about 105 calories (3.5 calories/minute)

If you walk at a brisk to very brisk pace (3.5 to 4 mph) on a flat surface
You'll burn about 120 calories (4 calories/minute)

If you walk at a very, very brisk pace (4.5 mph) on a flat surface
You'll burn about 135 calories (4.5 calories/minute)

If you walk uphill at a brisk pace (3.5 mph)
You'll burn about 180 calories (6 calories/minute)

Figures are estimates based on a 135-pound person, courtesy of the Cooper Institute for Aerobics Research.

Form Fundamentals

- Feet should be hip-width apart, toes pointed forward.

- Walk tall, keeping your head and chest up, shoulders back and abdominals tight; don't arch your back.

- Bend your arms at a 90-degree angle, keeping your elbows in.

- With each step, plant your heel on the ground and roll through to the ball of your foot, then push off with your toes.

- Pump your arms.

- Squeeze your buttocks as if you were trying to hold a dime between them.

- Inhale and exhale deeply and rhythmically.

On the following pages you'll find a four-week walking program designed to maximize the time spent on your feet. With this program, you'll be strengthening your heart and lungs while you burn serious calories. You'll develop those metabolism-boosting muscles and firm up your lower body. I'll also be teaching you a new technique for increasing the intensity of your walks so your benefits continue to grow.

Over the next four weeks you'll be doing three different types of Walking Workouts: Basic, Challenge and Interval/Hill. Each week the program will get a little more difficult. As your heart, your lungs and your legs build strength and endurance, you'll pick up your pace to burn maximum calories and challenge your body.

Each walking workout takes 30 minutes. If you're a beginner or extremely out of shape, you'll need to work up to this amount. Start by doing about 10 minutes a day four times per week. During Week 2 increase your time to 20 minutes per workout. By the third week you should be up to 30 minutes per workout. I've provided beginner options along with each workout.

If time is tight, you can break your workouts down into 10-minute quickies. But remember: Your ultimate goal is to do 30 minutes of *continuous* aerobic activity. That's the best insurance policy for your heart. If you enjoy the walking, feel free to add 5 or 10 minutes (or even more) to your walks. With every extra minute, you'll be turning back the clock!

While you don't need any fancy equipment to do my Walking Workout, proper footwear is essential, and I suggest investing in a good pair of walking shoes. Walking shoes are designed for proper heel-to-toe roll-through; most also offer cushioned insoles, which are better for your joints. A good fit and proper support also are crucial for minimizing stress on joints and avoiding injuries. Moisture-absorbing, cushioned socks (not cotton!) will help keep your feet comfy and blister-free. If you're going to be walking outside rather than on a treadmill, you'll need a watch with a second hand to help you time the various stages of each workout.

To get the most out of your Walking Workouts, be sure to practice good form. Your feet should be about hip-width apart, toes pointed straight ahead. Your arms are bent at a 90-degree angle, elbows in close to your sides. Keeping your chest up, your shoulders back and your abdominals pulled in tight, plant your heel on the ground and roll through to the ball of your foot, then push off with your toes. Squeeze your buttocks as if you were trying to hold a dime between them. For maximum calorie burn, really pump those arms. Remember: The more muscles you use, the more calories you lose! Pumping your arms also helps reduce the swelling in your fingers—a common side effect of walking or hiking.

One of the things that I like most about fitness walking is that it's a perfect way to get outside and explore the world. When you're walking, you see things like interesting architecture and beautiful gardens that you might otherwise miss in a car. A good, brisk walk can clear your head and soothe your nerves. If the weather permits, you also can get a valuable dose of vitamin D via sunshine. (Just be sure to protect your eyes and skin with sunglasses and a hat.)

All three of my Walking Workouts can be done either outside or on a treadmill. Remember: Bad weather isn't an excuse to skip a workout. Fat cells and heart attacks don't take crummy weather into consideration! If you don't have access to a treadmill, you can power-walk at a shopping mall on rainy days. Or try one of my "Denise Austin" videos, which are great for women over 40: "Blast Away 10 Pounds," "Xtralite: Beginner's Tone Up," "Low Impact Aerobics," "Denise Austin's Yoga Workout," "Fat-Burning Blast," "Totally Firm—A Complete Workout with Weights," or "Mat Workout Inspired by JH Pilates."

A jump rope and exercise videos are perfect tools to keep at home if

At-a-Glance 4-Week Schedule

WEEK 1
Day 1: Basic Workout
Day 2: Basic Workout
Day 3: Basic Workout
Day 4: Basic Workout

WEEK 2
Day 1: Basic Workout
Day 2: Basic Workout
Day 3: Challenge Workout
Day 4: Basic Workout

WEEK 3
Day 1: Basic Workout
Day 2: Challenge Workout
Day 3: Basic Workout
Day 4: Interval/Hill Workout

WEEK 4
Day 1: Challenge Workout
Day 2: Challenge Workout
Day 3: Basic Workout
Day 4: Interval/Hill Workout

you can't afford a large piece of equipment like a treadmill. And don't forget to tune in to my *Fit and Lite* show on Lifetime—it airs every weekday morning.

One caution: Walking can be addictive—but in a good way! Once you feel the "runner's high" (it isn't just for runners) and see the fabulous results (a slimmer waistline and firmer legs, to name two), you could get hooked. So lace up your walking shoes and let's get started!

BASIC TRIMWALK WORKOUT

The warm-up (5 minutes): Start by walking for 5 minutes at an easy, relaxed pace (about 2.5 to 3.2 mph) to warm up your muscles and loosen up your joints. This is the time to get your form and your posture down. (See Form Fundamentals, page 42).

The workout (20 minutes): Now that your muscles are warm, it's time to pick up the pace. Begin walking at a moderate to brisk pace—if you're on a treadmill, about 3.2 to 3.7 mph. Your stride should be comfortable. Pump your arms to get the blood flowing and your heart rate up. Continue at this pace for 20 minutes.

The cool-down (5 minutes): Finish with 5 minutes of easy walking (about 2.5 to 3.2 mph) to let your body return to its normal temperature.

> Easy or comfortable pace = 2.5–3.2 mph
> Moderate or brisk pace = 3.2–3.7 mph
> Fast walk or jog = 3.8–4.5 mph

Beginner option: If you're just starting out, modify this workout as follows: Begin with a 3-minute easy warm-up (about 2.5 to 3.2 mph), 6 minutes of moderate to brisk walking (about 3.2 to 3.7 mph), and a 2-minute easy cool-down (2.5 to 3.2 mph). After one week or as soon as you feel ready, extend the length of your workout by doing a 3-minute easy warm-up, 10 minutes of moderate to brisk walking, and a 2-minute easy cool-down. Keep increasing your time when you are ready, and before long you'll be up to the full 30 minutes. You know your own body, so go at a pace that works for you!

Treadmill option: Follow the above workout, but work carefully to maintain proper form. If you are unsteady, hold on with one hand and pump your other arm, changing arms every two minutes.

Keep It Interesting

Need some help making it through the whole 30 minutes? Here are a few ways to keep your workouts interesting.

Listen to music. Nothing is more inspiring than music with an upbeat tempo. Try Sousa and march along. Or pick a favorite pop song that makes you keep stepping. As your fitness level improves, don't forget to update your tunes. The faster the beat, the faster you'll walk!

Keep good company. Walk with a friend, family member or coworker. Talking as you walk helps pass the time and keeps you from looking at your watch. You'll go farther and faster as you focus on your buddy instead of your boredom. This is also a great way to socialize. Try joining a walking club or call a neighbor.

Open your eyes. If you're walking outdoors, keep your head up and take a look at the scenery—it's beautiful out there! Check out the gorgeous gardens, admire the architecture and absorb all the different colors. Listen to all the soothing sounds—birds chirping, children playing, leaves rustling.

Try a new route. We tend to be creatures of habit, but it's amazing how fast the time passes when you're exploring a new neighborhood or trail. Clock your new routes in the car so you know how much distance you're covering.

CHALLENGE WORKOUT

The warm-up (5 minutes): Start by walking for 5 minutes at an easy to moderate pace (2.7 to 3.5 mph) to warm up your muscles and loosen your joints.

The workout (20 minutes): When you've finished the warm-up, pick up the pace and start moving. You should be walking at a very brisk pace (about 3.5 to 4.5 mph). If you feel up to it, you may even want to try a slow jog. Either way, keep those arms pumping and don't be afraid to work up a sweat. Remember: This workout should be difficult enough that you feel challenged but not so difficult that you can't maintain your pace for the next 20 minutes. Your breathing should get heavier but you should still be able to engage in conversation. Never sacrifice form for speed—if you have to, move a little slower to keep proper form.

The cool-down (5 minutes): Return to an easy to moderate pace (2.7 to 3.5 mph) for your 5-minute cool-down. Allow your body to readjust, focus on your breathing and enjoy the euphoria of a great workout. Way to go!

Beginner option: Maybe the Basic Workout isn't quite challenging enough but the Challenge Workout is too much. Try this variation to get you started: Warm up for 5 minutes at an easy pace (2.7 to 3.2 mph), then walk for 5 minutes at a moderate pace (3.2 to 3.5 mph). For the next 10 minutes, kick it into high gear (3.5 to 4.2 mph or a light jog). Return to a moderate pace for 5 minutes (3.2 to 3.5 mph) before cooling down for 5 minutes at an easy pace (2.7 to 3.2 mph). If you can't sustain 10 fast minutes, then try varying your speed: 1 minute at a moderate pace followed by 1 minute at a fast pace. Continue alternating for 10 minutes.

Treadmill option: Instead of just speeding up, raise the incline on your treadmill. Try a 2- to 4-percent incline. For maximum calorie burn, pump with both arms. (In recent studies, women who had treadmills in their home and walked several times a day for short periods tended to lose the most weight and kept it off. So maybe a treadmill is a good investment for you.)

Challenge Change-Up

Experiment with different strides to add a challenging change to your workout.

Longer strides. Works the buttocks and the hips while stretching the calf muscles.

Shorter strides. Taking smaller, shorter steps allows you to move more quickly, so you can get your heart rate up higher. Like a race walker, try to get your powerful hips involved—and really pump those arms!

Uphill. Great for the backs of the legs and butt, as you use more muscle to climb.

Downhill. Equally effective, as you use your quads to control your body and fight the downward gravitational pull.

INTERVAL WORKOUT

The warm-up (5 minutes): Start by walking for 5 minutes at an easy to moderate pace (2.7 to 3.5 mph) to warm up your muscles and loosen your joints.

The workout (20 minutes): This is my favorite—it really revs up your metabolism! For the next 20 minutes you're going to alternate spurts of higher-intensity walking ("work") and lower-intensity walking ("rest"). You'll be timing yourself, so make sure you have a watch if you're walking outside. Start by doing 2 minutes of very brisk walking (about 3.5 to 4.5 mph) or jogging. Your goal is to get your heart rate up—you should be breathing hard enough that holding a conversation would be difficult. After 2 minutes slow down to an easy walk (about 2.7 to 3.5 mph); continue at this pace for 2 minutes, so you can catch your breath and lower your heart rate. Continue doing 2 minutes of very brisk walking followed by 2 minutes of easy walking until your 20 minutes is up. As you get more fit, you can vary the length of your intervals to increase the challenge—for instance, you can extend the high-intensity "work" portion of your interval to 3 or 4 minutes. Or you can reduce the lower-intensity "rest" interval to 1 minute.

Beginner option: Do 1 minute of high-intensity walking ("work") and 1 or 2 minutes of easy walking ("rest"). As you get in better shape, gradually lengthen the work portion of your intervals.

Treadmill option: Another way to increase the intensity of your workout is to raise the incline on your treadmill. During your warm-up and low-intensity "rest" intervals, keep the treadmill flat or at a 1 percent incline. During your high-intensity "work" intervals, raise it to anywhere from a 3- to a 12-percent incline. You may have to walk at a slower speed, but as long as your heart rate is elevated, you're in business. Continue raising and lowering the incline on the treadmill every 2 minutes for the entire 20-minute workout. This "hill" training is also great for toning the backs of your legs and buttocks.

Triathalon Cardio Workout Option

For a more advanced workout, why not combine low-impact activities such as walking, biking and swimming? Organize a competition among friends on a Saturday; walk a mile, swim 20 laps and then bike to a scenic destination for a picnic lunch. What do you know—you're a triathlete!

THE STRENGTH-TRAINING WORKOUT

Welcome to the wonderful world of strength training! Weight lifting is one of the best age-defying secrets around. You have over 640 different muscles to help you look toned, fit and young. The key is knowing how to use these age-stoppers. That's where I come in.

While many aerobic activities help strengthen your muscles (walking and running develop your leg muscles, for example), the fastest, most effective way to build metabolism-boosting muscle is by lifting weights. This form of strength training involves doing exercises to isolate and target specific muscles or muscle groups using weights for resistance. Not only will my weight-training workouts help ignite your metabolism and tone and tighten your muscles, they will improve your posture and balance and strengthen your bones to fight osteoporosis.

My muscle-building workout can be done either at home or in a gym. In terms of equipment, you'll need a set of 3-, 5-, 8- and 12-pound dumbbells. These hand weights can be purchased quite inexpensively at any major sporting goods store. If necessary, you can substitute soup cans, water bottles or other objects that you have lying around the house. But if you're serious about getting in shape—and I know that you are—I recommend investing in the real thing. For some exercises, you'll also need a sturdy chair and a small towel.

Since many of you may be new to weight lifting, we'll start out with relatively light weights. In the photos, I'm using 5-pound weights, but you may want to start with 3-pound weights, depending on your fitness level. (If you are a beginner, you should do the exercises once or twice without weights until you get the hang of them.)

When your muscles are no longer challenged, it's time to switch to a heavier weight. Your goal with each workout is to work your target muscle or muscle group to the point of fatigue. In other words, you want your triceps to feel tired during your last few triceps kickbacks. If you can't lift the weight one more time at the end of an exercise, you've reached fatigue. If this seems a bit extreme, rest assured that you don't have to kill yourself to gain benefits. But your aim is to get stronger, so try to keep those muscles challenged!

Each muscle-building exercise is divided into sets and repetitions (reps). A set consists of 8 to 12 reps. Every rep is a thoughtful, controlled movement. You're working your muscle through its full range of motion, contracting and releasing as you lift and lower. Even though it's tempting, don't rush. Moving too quickly or in a jerky, uneven way will minimize the benefits.

In this workout you'll be doing one to two sets of each exercise, depending on your fitness level. As you focus on the muscle that you're working, try to relax the rest of your body, including your face, neck and shoulders. If you're holding tension in other areas, your target muscles won't benefit as much as they should.

You've already heard me talk about breathing. But proper breathing is especially important in strength training. Here's a little rule of thumb: You should always exhale as you contract, or use, the muscle and inhale as you release, or relax, it. When you're doing abdominal exercises, improper breathing can actually negate some of the good you're doing—so follow the instructions carefully!

Each strength workout is designed to take about 30 minutes. But like many of my exercise programs, you can split it up into three 10-minute mini-workouts that you can sprinkle throughout your day. To make it easy for you, I've already divided each of the three routines into three parts. Now you can schedule your muscle building into your own timetable!

The exercises in each of the three workouts should be completed in the order shown. We save the lower back and ab moves for last, since these are the core muscles that stabilize your body for the upper and lower body exercises. If your core muscles are tired, you may be unable to work other parts of your body as effectively.

Stretching is very important after strength training—so be sure to give those pooped-out muscles a good stretch at the end of your workout. Research shows that stretching incorporated into a weight-lifting program can help you build strength faster. Don't forget to record the details of your workout in the Workout Log (page 110) to see your progress.

I bet you're wondering how long it will take before you see results. If you do your workouts three times a week, you should see noticeable improvement in three weeks or less. Look in the mirror to see the changes—firmer muscles, more definition, and an overall toned appearance. You'll also feel stronger and have more energy.

Here's what you'll need to get started:

- A set of 3-, 5-, 8- and/or 12-pound dumbbells
- A sturdy chair
- A small towel
- 1- to 3-pound ankle weights (optional)

Tips for Strength-Training Success

- Lift the weights in a slow, controlled manner.

- Use proper form—don't get sloppy!

- Move your muscles through a full range of motion.

- Squeeze your target muscle as you do each move.

- Muscles need 48 hours to repair themselves after a workout, so skip a day between strength-training sessions.

- Don't let your mind wander. If you focus your thoughts on the muscle you're working, you'll get better results and really feel all the good that you're doing for your body.

- If you can do all the reps easily, it's time to add weight.

- Stretch after each exercise or at the end of your workout.

WORKOUT #1

Upper Body

We rarely use our upper body muscles in popular aerobic activities like walking and biking, so chances are you have little strength in your top half. The good news is that it won't take long to get results. And to me, there's nothing more attractive than toned arms. Let's get lifting!

One-Arm Row. Holding a dumbbell in your right hand, stand with your feet apart as shown. Bend your knees slightly and keep your abdominals tight. Rest your left palm on your left thigh or use a chair or bench for support. Begin with your arm extended all the way down so you get a good stretch. Keeping your back flat, pull the weight up toward your armpit, then lower it. Do 8 to 12 reps. Then switch sides. When you're finished, do another set of 8 to 12 reps on each side for a total of two sets. *Benefits: Strengthens and tones your middle and upper back.*

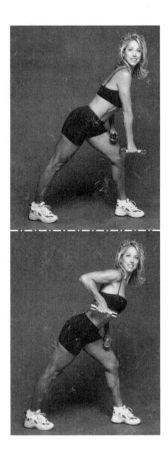
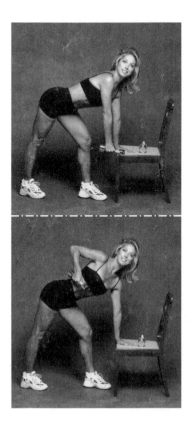
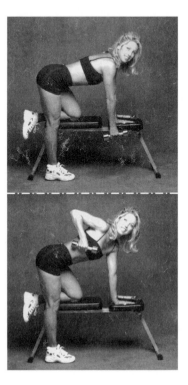

Triceps Kickback. Hold a dumbbell in your right hand and stand with your left leg in front of your right, left knee slightly bent. For support, rest your left hand on your left thigh or lean on a chair or bench. Keeping your abs tight and your back flat, raise your right elbow until the upper part of your arm is almost parallel with the floor; keep your elbow in close to your body. Straighten your right arm as shown. Be sure to squeeze your triceps (the back of your arm) as you straighten your arm. Return your right hand to the starting position. Do 8 to 12 reps, then switch sides and repeat. When you're finished, do another set of 8 to 12 reps on each side for a total of 2 sets.
Benefits: Strengthens the backs of your arms (triceps).

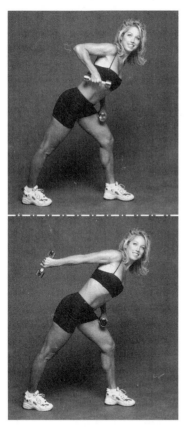
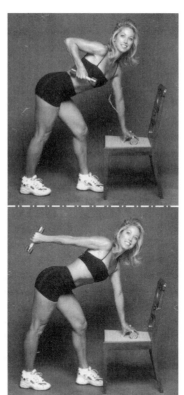
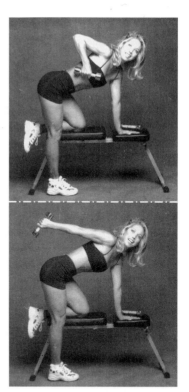

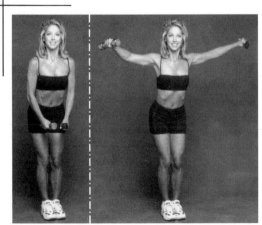

Side Raises. Stand with your feet shoulder-width apart, abs tight, back straight and knees slightly bent. Start with your hands at your sides as shown. Inhale as you lift your hands up to just above your shoulders, elbows bent only slightly. Exhale as you lower your hands back to your sides. Do 2 sets of 8 to 12 reps, resting briefly in between.
Benefits: Firms and tones the sides of your shoulders.

Lower Body

With every step we take, we're using our lower body muscles. Problem is, many of us use the same muscles over and over. The exercises below target a variety of muscles, including ones in your inner and outer thighs—traditional weak spots. End result: a toned, jiggle-free lower body. You'll look great in those "short shorts"!

Wide-Stance Squat. Stand with your feet wider than your shoulders, arms by your sides, toes turned out slightly (like second position in ballet). Bend your knees and slowly "sit back" to lower your buttocks toward the floor, keeping your body weight over your heels. Your thighs should be as close to parallel to the floor as possible. Squeeze your buttocks as you straighten your legs to return to the starting position. If you have a history of knee problems, begin with a partial squat, one quarter of the way down. Do 2 sets of 8 to 12 reps, resting briefly in between.
Benefits: Strengthens and tones your buttocks (gluteals) and inner thighs. For an advanced workout, hold a dumbbell in each hand.

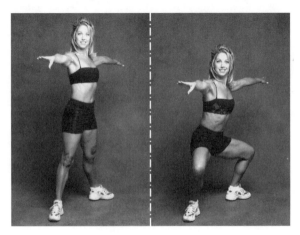

Hamstring Curls. In a standing position, slowly bend your left knee and extend your right leg behind you. Then slowly curl your right heel toward your buttocks. Be sure to keep your back straight, keep your abs tight and squeeze your buttocks together throughout the entire movement. Lower your right leg to the starting (straight leg) position. Do 2 sets of 8 to 12 reps on each side. Relax and repeat.
Benefits: Strengthens and tones the backs of your thighs (hamstrings).

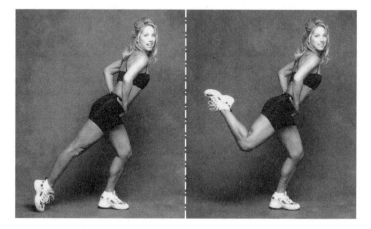

Outer Thigh Trimmer. Lie on the floor on your left side. Your head, shoulders and hips should form one straight line. Bend your left leg behind you, placing your right hand on the floor in front of you for balance. Keeping your right leg straight and your foot relaxed, slowly raise your leg. Lower it back to the floor, then repeat for 2 sets of 8 to 12 reps, resting briefly in between sets. Switch sides and repeat. Optional: Place 1- to 3-pound ankle weights on each ankle or hold the weight on your thigh.
Benefits: Strengthens and slims your outer thigh area.

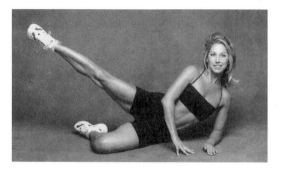
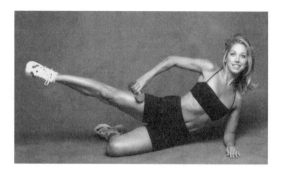

Abs/Lower Back

Yoga, Pilates and Tai Chi practitioners believe that all of our energy flows from our abdominals, our core. And there are plenty of other reasons to strengthen those middle muscles, including better posture and a healthy back. Strong abdominals and lower back muscles not only help you stand tall like a dancer and minimize love handles and the midlife bulge, they help guard against back pain, the number-one complaint among women over 40.

Ab Crunch. Lie on your back with your knees bent and your feet on the floor. Rest your head in your hands, keeping your neck and shoulders relaxed. Press your lower back firmly into the floor; there should be no arch in your back at all. Exhale as you contract your abdominals to slowly lift your shoulders and feet off the floor; focus on pressing your belly button toward your spine. This is a very small, controlled movement. Slowly lower your shoulders and feet to the floor. Do 2 sets of 8 to 12 reps, resting briefly between each. If you have neck problems, use a towel instead of your hands to hold your head.

Benefits: Strengthens and firms your main abdominal muscle (rectus abdominus).

Variation: For an added challenge, hold a 1- to 3-pound weight above your head.

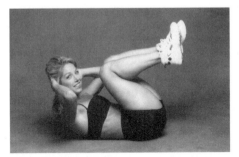

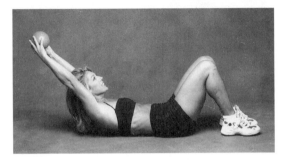

For an extra challenge

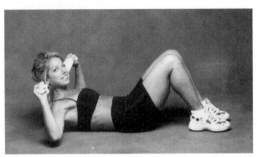

Easier on the neck

Lower Tummy Tightener. Lie on your back and place your hands palms down just beneath your buttocks. This allows you to keep your lower back flat on the floor during the exercise. Lift your legs off the floor, bend them slightly and cross your ankles. Exhale as you contract your abs to lift your bent knees toward your chest. Your knees should stay bent at the same angle throughout the entire exercise. Lower your legs slightly back down and repeat. This is a very short range of movement; your tailbone should lift off the floor only 3 to 5 inches. Do 2 sets of 8 to 12 reps, resting briefly between each set. If you have back problems, place a pillow beneath your lower back for comfort.

Benefits: Tightens and firms your lower abs—especially great if you've had a baby.

Variation: For an extra challenge that will also strengthen your inner thighs, squeeze a towel between your legs.

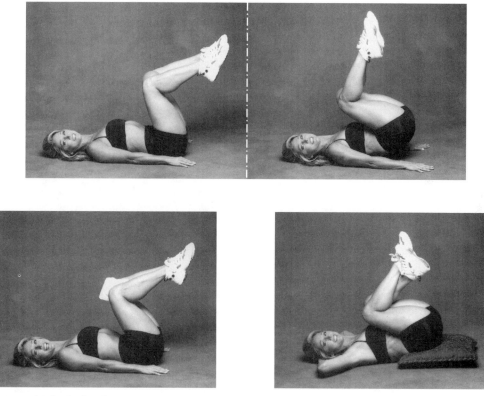

Inner-thigh challenge *Easier on the lower back*

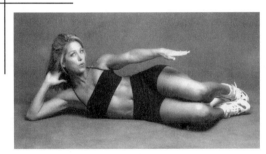

Oblique Curls. Lie on the floor on your right side with knees bent. Keep your back straight. There should be no arch in your back at all. Place your left hand out to the side and your right hand behind your head for support. Exhale as you lift your right shoulder blade off the floor, and tighten the sides of your waistline. Relax as you lower back to the floor. Slower is better. Do 2 sets of 8 to 12 reps, resting briefly between each set. Switch sides and repeat.

Benefits: Strengthens the inner and outer obliques (sides of your waist) to minimize those love handles.

Back Strengthener. Begin in a push-up position, with hands beneath your shoulders and abs tight. Pull one knee in and reach it slightly toward your opposite shoulder. Return to starting position. Repeat with opposite leg. Continue alternating legs for 8 to 12 reps.

Benefits: Strengthens and elongates your abdominals and strengthens your arm and back muscles.

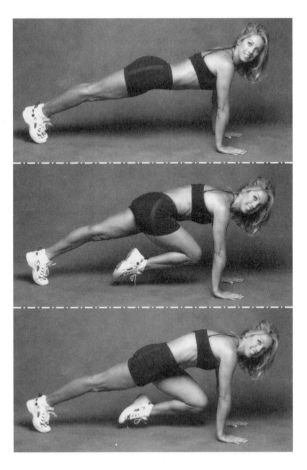

WORKOUT #2

Upper Body

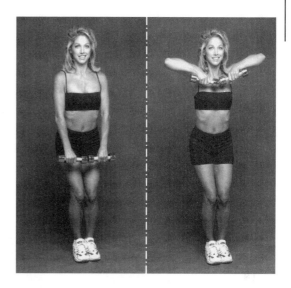

Upright Row. Hold two dumbbells in front of you with your palms facing in and stand with your knees slightly bent, abs tight. Inhale and squeeze your shoulder blades together as you raise the weights up toward your shoulders. Your arms should form a V shape, as shown. Exhale as you slowly lower your arms to starting position. Do 2 sets of 8 to 12 reps, resting briefly between each set.
Benefits: Strengthens and tones your upper back and shoulders.

Biceps Curls. Stand up tall with your knees slightly bent, back flat, abs tight. With an underhand grip, hold a dumbbell in each hand in front of your thighs. Exhale as you slowly raise the weights toward your upper arms and shoulders, bending your arms at the elbows. Be sure not to arch your back as you lift the weights, and keep your elbows close to your body throughout the movement. Hold momentarily, then return your hands to the starting position. Do 2 sets of 8 to 12 reps, resting briefly after each. You can also do this exercise sitting down.
Benefits: Tightens and tones the front of your arms (biceps).

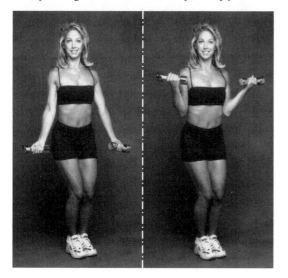

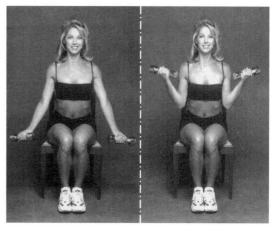

Exercise: Burn Back the Clock!

Chest Firmer (Pec Flies). Sit back on a chair or weight bench with your knees bent and your feet flat on the floor. Hold the dumbbells in your hands with your arms extended (arms straight but not locked in the elbow joint) at shoulder level above your chest, palms facing in. Slowly lower your arms out to the sides, keeping them bent at the same angle throughout the movement. Squeeze your chest as you slowly return your arms to the starting position. This can also be performed lying down on the floor. Do 2 sets of 8 to 12 reps, resting briefly between sets.

Benefits: Strengthens and firms your chest muscles (pectorals) for a better bustline.

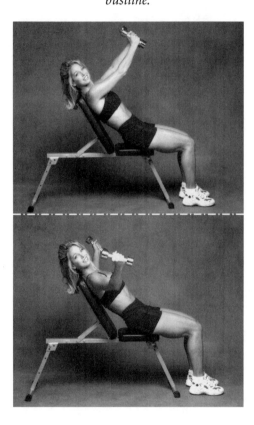 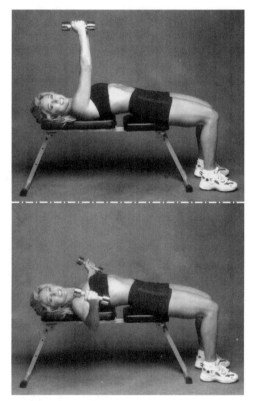

Lower Body

Basic Lunge. Stand with your feet together, then take a giant step forward with your right foot (you can hold on to a chair for balance). Keeping your weight over your back toes and your front heel, bend both knees to lower yourself toward the ground; your front knee should be directly above your ankle. Keep your back straight throughout the move. Straighten legs to return to a standing position. Do 2 sets of 8 to 12 reps, resting briefly between sets, then switch legs and repeat. If you have bad knees, modify this lunge by only bending your knees slightly—you're still firming those thighs.
Benefits: Works your entire leg, with an emphasis on your buttocks (gluteals) and the front of your thighs (quadriceps).

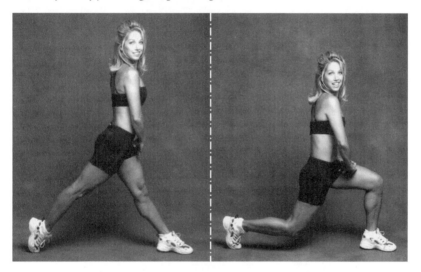

Inner Thigh Firmer. Lie on the floor on your left side. Your head, shoulders and hips should form a straight line. Keeping your legs straight, slowly raise your legs about 8 inches off the floor. Release your bottom leg down to the floor—then bring it back up to meet your top leg. Feel your inner thighs working on the "up" motion. Do sets of 8 to 12 reps, then switch sides and repeat.
Benefits: Tones and firms your inner thigh muscles.

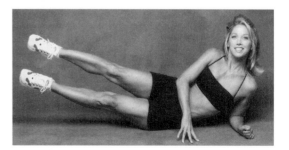

Bun Burner. On all fours, keep your back straight, hips square and abs tight. Raise your leg up, keeping it bent at a 90 degree angle. Your thigh should be parallel to the floor. Now cross it behind you over the other knee, then back to starting position. Do 2 sets of 8 to 12 reps, then switch legs.

Benefits: Firms and tightens the buns (gluteus maximus).

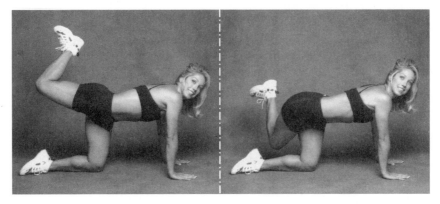

Calf Shaper. Stand with your feet hip-width apart and place your hands on your hips. Bend your left knee and place your left foot behind your right calf. Then lift your right heel up and down slowly. Do 2 sets of 8 to 12 reps, then switch legs.

Benefits: Firms, shapes and sculpts your lower legs (calves).

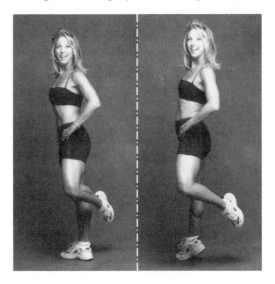

Total Tummy Tightener. Lying on your back, elevate your feet and place your hands behind your head. Lift your head and shoulders off the floor and at the same time "pulse" your hips up off the floor to also work the lower end of your abs. "Pulse" for 15–20 reps. Make sure the small of your back stays down against the floor.
Benefits: Strengthens and firms the entire rectus abdominis.

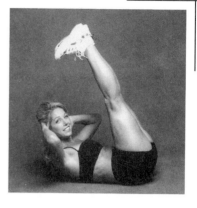

Bicycles. Lie on your back with your left leg straight up in the air and your right knee bent in toward your chest. Press your back firmly into the floor; there should be no arch in it at all. Rest your head in your hands, but keep your neck and shoulders relaxed. Exhale as you pull your right knee in toward your chest. At the same time, raise your left shoulder to meet your right knee. Straighten out your right leg and return your left shoulder to its normal position. Then draw your left leg in toward your chest to touch your right elbow. Continue to alternate sides, as if you're riding a bicycle. Keep the movement smooth and flowing; try to keep your feet from touching the floor. Do 2 sets of 8 to 12 reps, resting briefly between sets (one rep equals one twist on each side).
Benefits: Strengthens and tones your inner and outer obliques (sides of your waist) for a sexy, hourglass figure.
Variation: For a more advanced workout, keep your feet closer to the floor. The lower the legs, the more intense the workout.

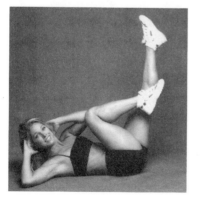 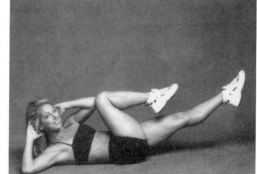

Low Hover. Start in a modified straight-legged push-up position with elbows on the floor directly below your shoulders, hips lifted slightly and abs tight. Elongate your abs and back by lifting your pelvis and hold for 30 seconds. Rest and repeat. Focus on the "core" of your body, your torso and abs.

Benefits: Strengthens and lengthens your abdominal muscles as well as the back extensors (middle and upper back muscles).

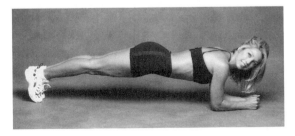

Back Strengthener. Kneel on all fours, knees directly below your hips and hands beneath your shoulders. Simultaneously extend your right leg and your left arm. Hold for 8–10 seconds. Focus on keeping your back flat and buttocks squeezed. Relax and repeat with opposite leg and arm. Continue alternating two more times.

Benefits: Strengthens the entire back muscle (erector spinae).

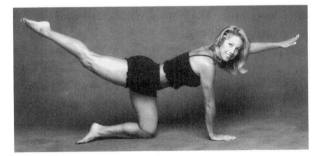

WORKOUT #3

Upper Body

Upper Back Firmer. Holding a dumbbell in each hand, sit on a chair with your feet flat on the floor. Lean forward so that your chest is near your thighs. Squeeze your shoulder blades together as you slowly lift your arms straight out to the sides, leading with your pinky fingers. Return to the starting position. Make sure that the movement is slow and deliberate; don't swing the weights. Do 2 sets of 8 to 12 reps, resting briefly between sets.

Benefits: Strengthens and firms your upper back muscles—no more bra overhang!

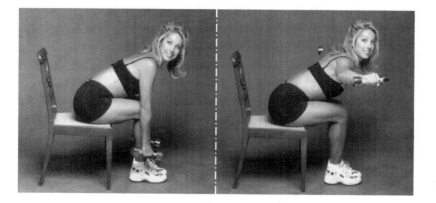

Triceps Dip. Place your hands on the edge of a sturdy chair or weight bench, fingers facing toward you, knees bent, feet flat on the floor. Shift your buttocks forward so they're in front of the chair. Bend your elbows to slowly lower your buttocks toward the floor, keeping your back straight and close to the chair. Straighten your arms to lift your buttocks back up to chair height, feeling the workout in the backs of your arms. You can also do this exercise using the edge of a bench, a couch or a bed. Repeat 8 to 10 times.

Benefits: Strengthens and tones the backs of your arms (triceps) to combat upper arm jiggle.

Variation: For a more advanced exercise, extend one leg straight out in front of you as you lower your buttocks to the floor.

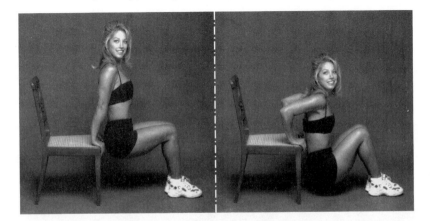

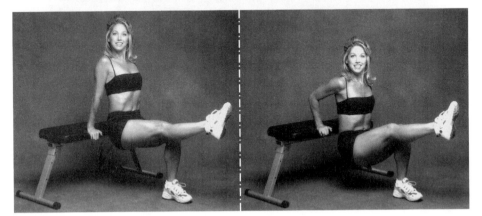

Chest Press. Lie back in a chair or on a weight bench with your knees bent and your feet flat on the floor. Holding a dumbbell in each hand, slowly bend your arms so that your elbows are parallel to your shoulders. Push the weights straight up so that your arms are extended directly over your chest, keeping your lower back pressed firmly into the bench. Avoid locking your elbows at the top of the movement. Slowly lower to the starting position. Do 2 sets of 8 to 12 reps, resting briefly between sets. You can also do this exercise lying on the floor.
Benefits: Strengthens and firms your chest muscles (pectorals).

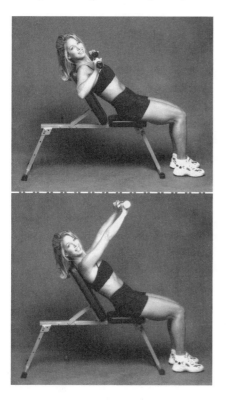

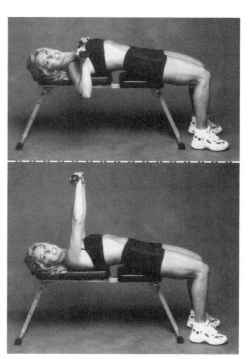

Overhead Press. Hold a dumbbell in each hand and sit on a chair with your abs tight and your back straight. Start with your hands at your shoulders. Exhale as you raise your hands over your head. Inhale as you slowly lower the weights back down to your shoulders. Do 2 sets of 8 to 12 reps, resting briefly between sets.

Benefits: Sculpts your shoulders for a beautiful look and better posture.
Variations: Standing, bend your left knee and extend your right leg back in a lunge position, raising and lowering the weights over your head. Or, remain sitting, but alternate your arms rather than raising both at the same time.

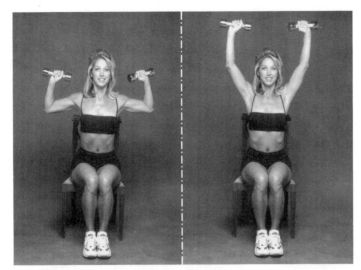

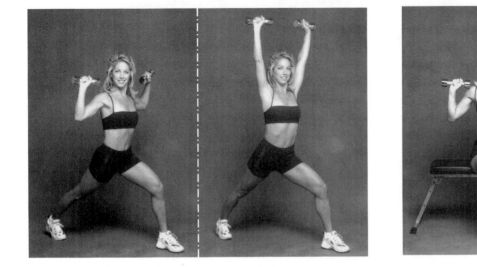

Lower Body

Bottoms Up. Lie on your back with your knees bent, feet flat on the floor, arms by your sides. Squeeze your buttocks and tighten your abdominals as you lift your buttocks off the floor (3 to 6 inches) by tilting your pelvis up. Hold for a few seconds, then lower your bottom down one vertebra at a time. For better results, place a towel between your knees. Do 2 sets of 8 reps, resting briefly between sets.
Benefits: Strengthens and lifts your buttocks (gluteals) for a great rear view.
Variation: For a more advanced exercise, straighten and lower one leg while holding your pelvis up.

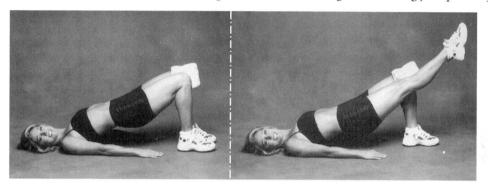

Power Squat. Extend your arms and stand with your feet a little wider than hip-width apart, arms outstretched, parallel to the floor. Bend your knees and slowly "sit back" to lower your buttocks toward the floor, keeping your body weight over your heels. Your thighs should be as close to parallel to the floor as possible. Squeeze your buttocks as you straighten your legs to return to the starting position. If you have a history of knee problems, begin with a partial squat, one quarter of the way down. Do 2 sets of 8 to 12 reps, resting briefly between sets.
Benefits: Strengthens and tones your buttocks (gluteals) and thighs.

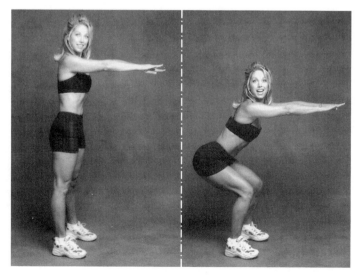

Exercise: Burn Back the Clock!

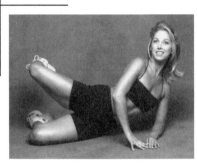

Hip Slimmers. Lie on your left side on a carpet or a mat. Raise your torso and support yourself on your left forearm. Bend both legs. Keep abs tight while you raise the top leg up and down (about 8 to 12 inches). Slowly return it to the floor. Do 1 set of 16 to 24 reps with each leg.
Benefits: Strengthens and tones your outer thigh and hip muscles.

Inner Thigh Toner. Lie on your side, lift up your top leg and hold it in place. Then lift and "pulse" the bottom leg toward the top leg. Pulse 5 times and then lower leg. Switch sides and repeat.
Benefits: A great way to tone and firm up your inner thighs (adductor muscles).

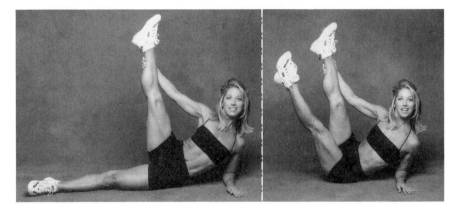

Abs/Lower Back

Waistline Trimmer. Lie on your back with your hands behind your head. Elevate your feet. If your hamstrings are too tight, bend your knees. Use your abdominals to lift your chest and your left shoulder off the floor slightly and twist the left elbow toward your knee. Do 2 sets of 8 reps to one side, then switch. Concentrate on one side of the waistline at a time. Keep feet flexed.
Benefits: Strengthens your obliques (the sides of your waistline).

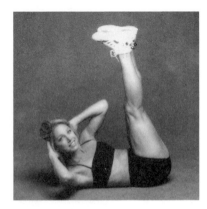

Lower Ab Strengthener. Lie on your back with your knees bent out to the sides and the soles of your feet together. Press the small of your back to the floor as you use your abdominals to lift your feet (6 to 8 inches), head and shoulders off the floor. Hold for 3 to 5 seconds before lowering. Keep your abs tight as you focus on "pressing your belly button in." Relax and repeat 10 times.
Benefits: Strengthens lower abs and pelvic floor muscles.

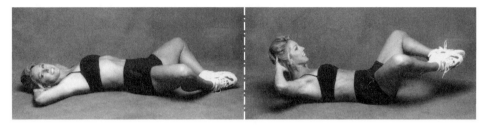

Reverse Crunch. Lie on your back with one knee bent at a 90-degree angle and the other extended straight up into the air, keeping your feet flexed and your hands behind your head. With your back pressed to the floor, exhale as you use your lower abdominals to gently lift your hips off the floor, pressing your belly button in toward your spine. With your hips raised, pull your bent knee in as close to your chest as possible, keeping the other leg straight up. This is a very small movement; your knee should stay bent at the same angle throughout the move. Inhale as you release and lower your hips to the floor. Relax and repeat with the other leg. Alternate legs for a total of 15 reps.
Benefits: Strengthens the lower abs.

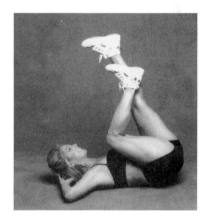

Spine Strengthener. Lie facedown with your arms folded under your chin. Keep your hips pressed firmly down as you lift your legs about 4 to 8 inches off the floor; don't overarch your back. Squeeze your buttocks as you hold for 10 seconds. Release, then repeat. Do two or three times.
Benefits: Strengthens and sculpts your lower back as well as your buttocks (gluteals) and backs of your thighs (hamstrings).

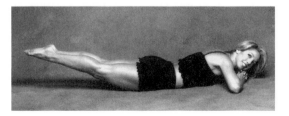

THE FLEXIBILITY AND BALANCE WORKOUT

Flexibility and balance don't have to dwindle as we age. By incorporating my yoga exercises and mat workout based on the Pilates method into your weekly routine, you can regain and even enhance these healthy body essentials.

Yoga, an ancient practice that developed 5,000 years ago in India, was once confined to small yoga studios. Now this popular workout can be found in gyms and health clubs across the country. Yoga is a series of controlled movements or "poses" with an emphasis on breathing and balance. It increases flexibility and balance, builds strength, relieves stress and fills your body with energy. This workout conditions your muscles without stress to your joints. Many people who find other forms of exercise uncomfortable have found yoga a soothing and enjoyable outlet. Some credit it for everything from curing their back pain to improving their golf game.

Developed by Joseph Pilates in the early twentieth century, Pilates (pronounced puh-LAH-teez) quickly became a favorite workout of dancers. Today it's moving into the mainstream as *the* exercise of Hollywood celebrities. Pilates is a series of movements that places intense concentration on particular muscle groups, especially the abdominals. They can be done either on a mat or a special machine called a Reformer. Pilates improves posture, balance, muscle tone and mental stimulation. With Pilates you develop a lean, toned dancer's body by lengthening your muscles as you strengthen them.

It's great to have better balance and flexibilities since it can help you minimize aches and stiffness, increase your agility and improve your posture so you look taller and thinner. Flexibility—how far your muscles can extend—is crucial for balance, especially as we age. Moving with ease and confidence makes you feel and look better and can open up a window of opportunities. The end result is that your life will be more fulfilling, enjoyable and pain free.

For some of you, the benefits of this workout may not be as obvious as they are with your strength workouts. You may not be able to look in the mirror and see the muscles lengthening, but you should notice more energy and better circulation almost immediately—and over time you should experience dramatic improvements in range of motion and mobility. One of my friends, who is 57, thought her arthritis would never improve, but it has with the help of my yoga and Pilates-based moves. While weight training mainly targets large muscle groups like your buttocks and your thighs, the exercises on the following pages work smaller, deeper ones—the muscles needed to keep your body steady when walking on an icy sidewalk and, most important, keep your back healthy. Remember: Your spine is your lifeline. As you lengthen and strengthen your muscles, you'll improve your circulation and whisk tension out of your body. Each little workout will leave you feeling calm, balanced and rejuvenated. I recommend that you alternate the routines I've presented here: Do the yoga routine one day and the Pilates-based routine the next, and supplement the workouts with the other stretches I've included here to help specific problem areas, such as the hips and back.

This flexibility/balance routine is meant to be smooth and soothing, so eliminate any potential distractions before beginning. Turn off the television or radio. If you like, put on some soft music. Clear your mind of all thoughts. This isn't easy, I know. We are all so busy that our minds race constantly. But try to keep your mind in the moment for the next 5 to 10 minutes. Concentrate on your breathing and relax every part of your body. If your mind returns to thoughts of your grocery list, push it aside by focusing on your breathing. Let's make these next few minutes count!

These types of exercises may be new to many of you, so take your time and don't get discouraged. Practice makes perfect! As you do each move, be sure that your body stays in proper alignment; don't get sloppy. Each movement should be smooth and controlled. If you find yourself wobbling or falling over, try focusing on an item directly in front of you (a lamp, a light switch, a painting), tightening your abdominals and lengthening your breath. Remember: Quality is more important than quantity, so opt for a single good stretch over 10 halfhearted ones.

As you move through the postures, deep breathing will help draw your mind into the present. With the Pilates Method you inhale deeply through your nose and exhale through your mouth. In yoga your goal is to breathe in and out through your nose. Notice your belly expand as you draw air into your body and then flatten as you release it. Your breathing will help promote better concentration, so you can focus on getting the most out of each posture.

Once you learn these exercises, try to flow from one to the next without stopping. This will help boost your metabolism and pump blood to your joints and muscles. Every one of these moves originates at your core (your entire torso area, including your abs and back muscles), so keep your tummy active and engaged throughout each exercise. If you lose your balance, contract and tighten those abs—it will help you regain stability. As you go from one move to the next, try to elongate and lengthen your spine; this will help keep your backbone flexible and healthy.

As you do this workout, pay attention to the signals that your body is sending. Notice where you are holding your tension. (Are you hunching your shoulders? Clenching your jaw?) These exercises are designed to teach you how to tune in to your body. I want you to be aware of how your body feels every day. That way, if something *does* go wrong, you'll know it right away.

While you may be tempted to skip this part of my Stop the Clock program, DON'T. You'll be spending only 5 to 10 minutes on this workout, but the rewards are endless. Practice some of these moves each day if you can. I like to do them first thing in the morning, since they make me feel so good all day. Right before bed is another great time—it helps your mind relax and prepares your body for sleep. One friend of mine walks in the door from work and immediately takes 10 minutes to do these moves—an excellent way to forget the negative thoughts of the day. Find what works for you.

Height Enhancer: Grow an Inch Instantly

Whether you're doing a yoga move or sitting in front of a computer, proper posture is essential for preventing injury and rounded shoulders as you grow older. When you sit or stand tall, you breathe better and minimize the stress on your back and neck that can cause fatigue and headaches. With practically no effort, you can look five pounds slimmer and up to an inch taller! Many of you may be so used to slouching that you've forgotten what good posture feels like. Here's a great exercise to remind you.

Sit or stand in a comfortable position. Press your shoulders down and together as you lengthen your neck. Pretend there's a string attached to the top of your head pulling your body straight up. Relax your neck and shoulder muscles. Your rib cage should be lifted, not collapsing into your hips. There should be space between each and every vertabra. Feel your body growing taller!

YOGA WORKOUT

Palm Tree. Stand with your feet close together. Walk your left hand down the side of your leg, reaching as far down with your fingertips as is comfortable. Extend your right arm up and out over your head, palm facing down. Hold for 10 seconds and repeat on the other side. Try 3 sets. This stretch elongates the entire side of the body, opens up the hip and strengthens through the trunk (abs and back).

Variation: Lean over with left hand extending up and out over head, and your right arm bent at the elbow reaching behind you, palm facing out with fingertips walking up your spine between your shoulder blades. Hold 10 seconds and repeat on the other side.

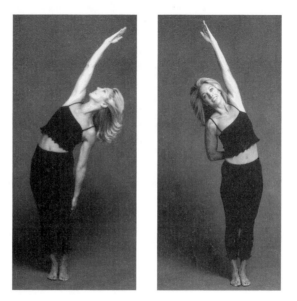

Eagle Pose. Stand with one leg behind the other. Wrap your arms around each other so that the palms eventually touch with thumbs hooked together and fingertips aligned. Pull your elbows away from the body to feel this stretch across your upper back. Twist to the side and flex the back leg. Hold for 15 seconds and repeat to the other side. This feels great for your shoulders, back and chest.

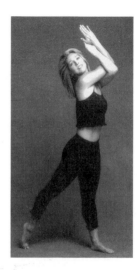

Exercise: Burn Back the Clock!

Camel. Place your hands on your lower back for support, with finger-tips facing down. Press your hips and pelvis forward while arching your back, very gently without going too far. This lean back always begins at the tailbone, never at the point of the lower back. Squeeze those buttocks for extra back support. Your chest and neck open up and your head falls back for a frontal body stretch and a spinal strengthener. Stay in this arch position for about 10 seconds and breathe through the stretch.

Variation: An easier version can be done on your knees.

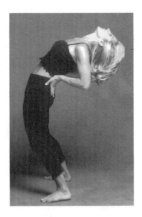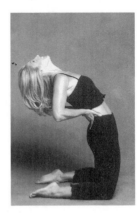

Warrior Pose. First, stand with your hands on your hips; step your feet apart so your ankles are in line with your wrists (your feet will be about 3 to 4 feet apart). Turn your left foot out at a 90-degree angle so your toes point directly to the left and rotate your right foot so your toes point to the left at a 45-degree angle. Bend your left knee as close as you can to a 90-degree angle (knee is directly over your ankle). Keeping your right leg straight, rotate your upper body so you're facing left. Push into your right heel. Look straight ahead or upward slightly. Then, extend both arms over your head, palms facing each other and fingers pointing toward the ceiling. Focus your eyes on your hands. Hold pose for 3 breaths. Return to standing position and repeat on the other side.

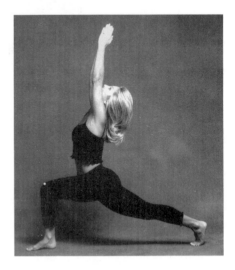

Triangle Pose. Stand with your legs 3 or 4 feet apart. Extend arms straight out to the sides at shoulder height, palms facing down. Turn your right foot out, away from your body, as in first position in ballet. Keeping your left leg straight, bend your right leg, resting your right arm on your right thigh for support. To give your neck a good stretch, turn your head to look at the ceiling. Take 3 deep breaths. Return to starting position and repeat on opposite side.

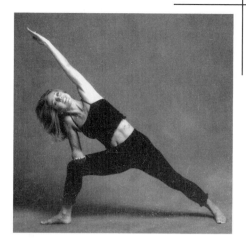

Forward Bend. Spread feet a little wider than shoulder-width apart. Keep a soft bend in your knees. Bend forward from the hip joints, extending your tailbone into the air, and stretch the spine out from that point. This pose relieves back tension. Your goal is flattening your back and then leaning forward. You can use a prop (a block or a chair) if you are starting out. Later, try to reach the floor. Hold this for 15 to 20 seconds, working up to a minute over time with practice.

Variation: Keep the feet together, lean over to a forward bend and roll onto the balls of the feet and back to the heels. Roll about three times forward and back to strengthen the ankles, achilles, calves and hamstrings.

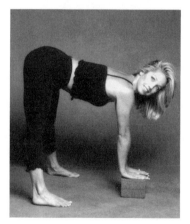
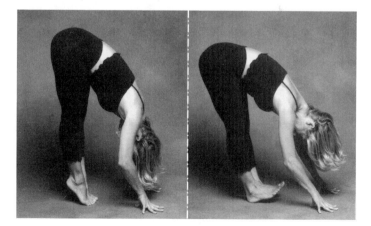

Standing Spinal Twist. Begin with feet wider than shoulder-width apart, feet pointing forward. A soft bend in the knees to alleviate too much tension in the hamstrings is fine. Bend forward, reaching your left arm toward the floor and reaching your right arm straight up over your head. Hold this for 10 seconds, then slowly come back to standing position and repeat on the other side.

Variation: A more advanced spinal twist is to reach through the legs with the right arm, wrapping up and around toward your rear and lower back. Allow the left arm to also wrap around the waist to the lower back, your goal being to meet the hands and hold this deep stretch for 15 seconds. You'll feel an opening into your left shoulder and through the rib cage/waistline area.

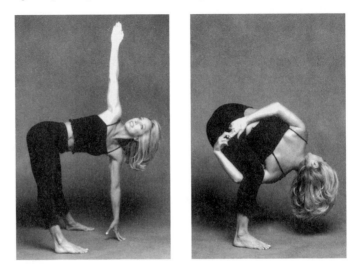

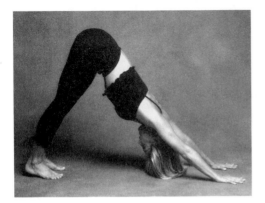

Downward-Facing Dog. Kneel on all fours, with your knees directly below your hips, hands slightly in front of your shoulders. Keeping your palms planted on the floor, lift your hips and buttocks up toward the ceiling until your legs are straight. Imagine that you're pointing your tailbone up toward the ceiling; your body should form an inverted V. Now, try to slowly and gently press your heels down, feeling the stretch in your calves. Hold the pose, as shown, for three deep breaths. Return to kneeling position, then repeat twice.

Cat Stretch. This is a great way to strengthen your abs and keep your back flexible. Kneel on all fours, being careful not to let your belly sag. Inhale as you keep your back flat, chin and chest lifted slightly upward. Now exhale as you slowly roll up your back, pull in your belly button and tighten your abdominal muscles. Do 3 complete sequences, inhaling and exhaling deeply.

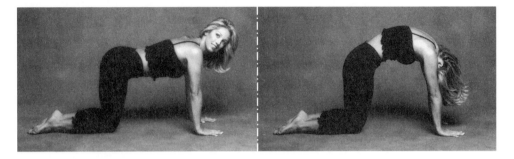

Child's Pose. Start in an upright kneeling position. Sit back on your heels. Keeping your buttocks on your heels, slowly bend forward and lower your head to the floor until you're curled up like a sleeping child, your forehead resting on the floor, arms by your sides, palms facing up. Take five deep breaths—and relax! This pose is designed to rejuvenate and nurture.

Variation: Extend your arms in front of you, palms facing down as you lower your head to the floor.

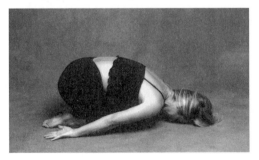 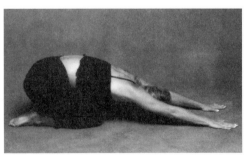

MAT WORKOUT INSPIRED BY THE PILATES METHOD

The Hundred (Beginner). Lie on your back, then pull your knees into your chest and place your arms over your head. Gently pull your chin forward to lift your head, neck and shoulder blades off the floor. Bring your arms down so your fingers are reaching toward your toes. Lift your arms 2 to 3 inches off the floor, then quickly pump (or pulse) your arms up and down. Breathe, inhaling for 5 counts and exhaling for 5 counts. Do this 5 times.

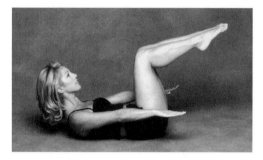

The Hundred (Advanced). Same as the beginner version, with one exception: Your legs should be extended straight up into the air, then lowered to the floor as much as possible while keeping your spine pressed against the floor and your belly flat. Hold this pose while you pulse with a count to 100.

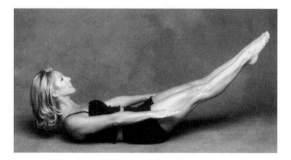

The Roll-Up. Start by lying on your back with your arms stretched over-head. Engage your abdominal muscles as you slowly roll your upper body up and forward into an upright position, lifting your arms toward the ceiling. Now, slowly continue reaching, with your arms curling over your fingertips toward your toes. Focus on using your abs. Your spine creates a C curve in the lower back by pulling your navel "in." Now slowly roll back down, one vertebra at a time. Relax and repeat twice.

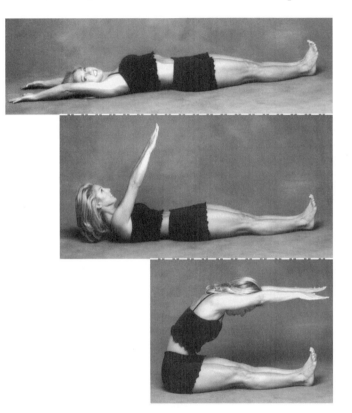

Bridge. Lie on the floor on your back with your knees bent, feet flat on the floor directly under your knees. Your knees should be hip-width apart. Lift your hips straight up so your body is supported by your shoulders and feet. Make sure your shoulders are pulled down and your neck is relaxed. Hold for 10 seconds. Lower and repeat. (Use caution if you have a bad neck.)

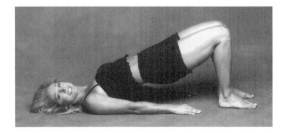

Exercise: Burn Back the Clock!

Single Leg Circles. Lie on your back, arms comfortably by your sides, legs extended straight. For a little stretch, hug your right knee into your chest, then straighten your leg so it extends up, forming a right angle with your body. Lower your right foot to your left side (like a windshield wiper), then swing it down until it's about 6 inches from your left leg. Continue swinging it (as if you're tracing an oval shape) back up toward the ceiling. The rest of your body should remain stable on the floor. The focus is to use your "power house" (abs) to create the circle with your leg. Repeat the circle 5 times. Reverse the direction and repeat 5 more times. Switch legs and repeat. (If you have any hip problems, do these carefully and stop if there's any pain.)

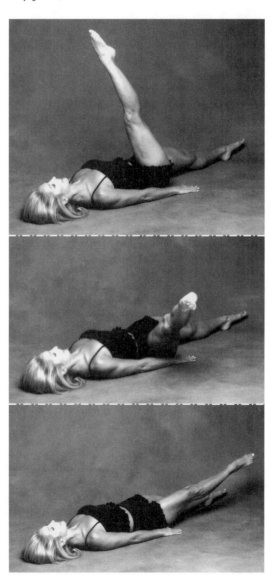

Rolling Like a Ball. Sit up with your knees bent in front of you, your buttocks as close to your heels as possible. Grasp your lower legs or ankles with both hands and "hug" them. Bring your chin in toward your chest, pulling your abs in and curving your back. Your body is curled up like a ball; your spine forms a C shape. Arch your feet so only your toes touch the floor. Inhale slowly as you roll back until your shoulder blades touch the floor, pulling your belly button into your spine. Exhale slowly as you roll back up to a seated position, maintaining a ball position. Repeat 6 times.

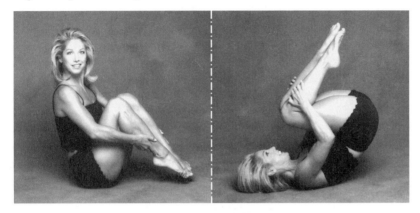

Single Leg Stretch. Lie on your back, legs extended in front of you, arms by your sides, palms facing down. Inhale slowly and tighten your abs as you bring your chin toward your chest, lifting your head and shoulders off the floor. Simultaneously bring your left (bent) knee into your chest. Place your left hand on your left ankle and your right hand on the inside of your left knee. Relax your shoulders and open your elbows out to the sides. Gently lift and hold your left knee to your chest for a count of 3, keeping your shoulders square and your torso stable. Switch legs and repeat, alternating 10 times. If you have neck problems, place a pillow under your neck and shoulders for support.

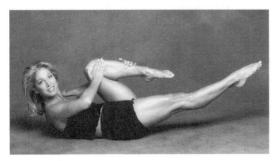
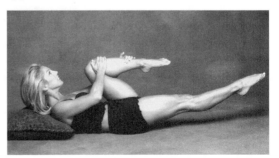

Exercise: Burn Back the Clock!

Double Leg Stretch. Begin by lying on your back with both knees pulled into your chest. Inhale and stretch your body long, pushing your legs straight in front of you and extending your arms over your head. Keeping your lower back and shoulders flat on the floor, reach your chin toward your chest, simultaneously raising your arms up until they're even with your ears. Exhale as you sweep your arms around by your sides. Use your abs as you slowly draw your legs toward your chest; hug your knees and hold. Tighten your abs as you stretch your limbs away from your torso. Pull limbs back in again, then hug your knees and hold. Repeat 3 to 6 times.

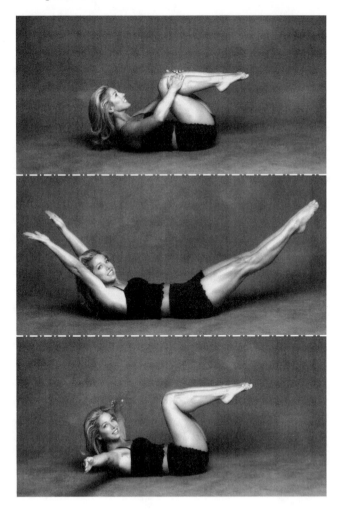

Crisscross. Lie on your back. Pull your knees into your chest and pull your chin forward. Rest your head in your hands. Lift your upper body (your head, neck and shoulders) off the floor. Exhale as you extend your left leg out straight while twisting your left elbow toward your right knee. Inhale as you return to center and switch. Repeat, this time extending your right leg out straight and twisting with your right elbow. Continue alternating legs 12 times total (6 on each side). Rest and repeat one more set.

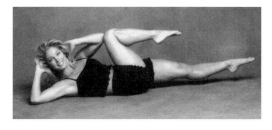

Spine Stretch Forward. Sit up with your legs extended in front of you, feet shoulder-width apart. Extend your arms in front of you as if you're sleepwalking. Tighten your abs as you lengthen your spine and lift your chest. Starting with your head, roll your upper torso down as you pull your abdominal muscles in. Keeping your arms elevated and your buttocks firm against the floor, continue rolling down until your spine forms a C (as if you're rounding yourself over a beach ball). Exhale. Inhale as you roll back up and sit tall. Exhale. Repeat 3 times.

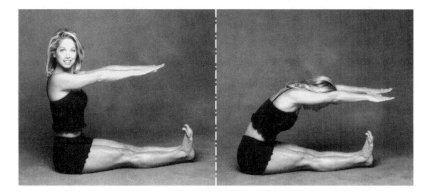

The Saw. Sit with your legs extended in front of you, feet shoulder-width apart, kneecaps pointing directly up toward the ceiling. Extend your arms out to the sides (you should be able to see your hands out of the corners of your eyes). Tighten your abs and lift your chest. Keeping your buttocks firmly planted on the floor, use your abs as you twist slowly to the right. Twist from your waist, not from your hips. Reach your left pinky finger toward your right baby toe. Then, leaning forward, stretch your torso toward your right leg. Your head should reach over your right knee. Relax your neck and keep your opposite hip down. Exhale slowly as you pulse 3 times (pretending to saw your baby toe off). Feel the stretch in your waist. Tighten your abs as you straighten up and return to center. Switch sides and repeat. Do 3 times total on each side.

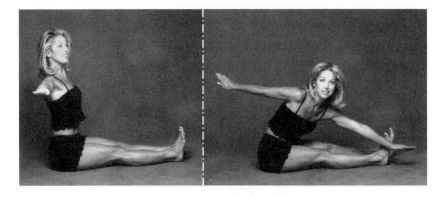

Seated Spine Twist. Sit with your legs extended in front of you and your arms extended straight out to the sides. Tighten your abs as you lift your chest and pull your shoulders down. Inhale as you slowly twist from your waist (not your hips) to the right as far as possible. Keep your eyes focused on your right hand as you shift it behind your body; your left hand comes forward. Both arms should form a straight line from front to back. Exhale as you twist back to the starting position. Repeat, this time twisting to the left side. Continue alternating twists, for a total of 3 times on each side.

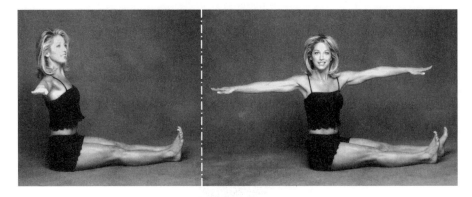

T-Stand Twist. Sit on your left hip with your legs slightly bent and your left hand on the floor directly under your shoulder. Pushing up on your left hand, inhale as you lift your hips off the floor and straighten your legs to create a straight line from your head to your toes, keeping your abs and buttocks tight and your shoulders relaxed. Lift your right arm up over your head to form the letter T. Hold for 10 to 15 seconds. Exhale as you lower your hips and bring your right arm back down to your side. Do 2 times, then switch sides and repeat.
Variation: For a simpler beginner variation, support yourself on one knee.

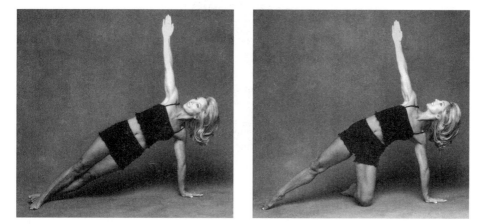

Teaser (Advanced). Lie on the floor on your back with your legs straight and your arms extended overhead. Inhale as you lift both legs while raising both arms overhead and in front of you until your fingers are pointed toward your toes. Your entire body should form a V, with your weight balanced on your buttocks. Keep your legs extended in the air as you exhale and slowly roll your upper body back down to the floor, vertabra by vertebra, and return your arms to an overhead position. Repeat 3 times.

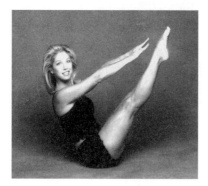

Exercise: Burn Back the Clock!

Swimming (Advanced). Lie on your belly with your legs straight, feet hip-width apart and slightly turned out, arms extended out straight over your head, palms facing down. Place your body weight over your pelvis and lower ribs, press your belly button toward your spine and elongate your neck, keeping your shoulders down and relaxed. Simultaneously lift your right arm and your left leg a few inches off the floor. Repeat, this time lifting your left arm and right leg. Do a total of 10 reps, alternating. Be sure to squeeze your buttock muscles so you don't overarch your lower back.

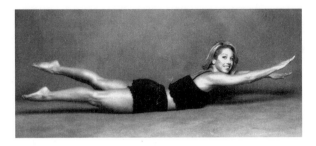

KEEP YOUR BACK HEALTHY IN 5 MINUTES A DAY

Back pain ranks second to the common cold as the most frequent medical complaint—and your risk increases as you get older. One of my good walking buddies, age 49, was recently diagnosed with degenerative disc disease, arthritis and a bone spur in her back. She had been very active, and the pain was intense. The doctor put her on steroids and recommended physical therapy, which did do some good. I also gave her some back exercises, and they've helped strengthen her back muscles.

As you get older, it's crucial to keep your spine strong and healthy. Consisting of small bones or vertebrae separated by cushy discs that act as shock absorbers, your spine is literally your lifeline, protecting the millions of nerves that control our everyday actions and agility. By strengthening and stretching the back and abdominal muscles that support the vertebrae with exercises like the ones shown on the following pages, you'll form a girdle of support that can help prevent pain and injuries, as well as stooped shoulders, as we age. These moves work your back muscles in four different ways—sideways (lateral flexion), forward (flexion), backward (extension) and rotationally—to keep it strong and supple. For best results, do these exercises every day—they take only a couple of minutes! As you do them, try to focus on keeping your body relaxed and in a straight line. (If you have a bad back, be sure to check with your doctor first.)

Spinal Twist (Back Rotation). Sit on the floor with your legs extended in front of you, feet flexed. Bend your right knee, then lift your right foot up and place it on the left side of your left knee. Bending your left arm, place your left elbow on the outside of your right knee and turn your upper body to the right. Try to keep your shoulders down as you twist your spine farther to the right. Pushing your chest forward will further lengthen your spine. Hold the pose for three deep breaths. Return to starting position and repeat on opposite side.

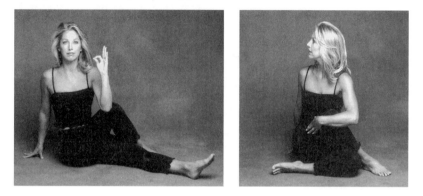

Forward Bend (Flexion). Sit on the floor with your legs extended straight in front of you. Keeping your back straight and your abdominals pulled in, reach both hands toward your toes as far as possible; hold the stretch for 15 to 30 seconds. Feel a gentle stretch all the way from your hamstrings to the top of your neck. As you stretch, you'll be increasing blood flow to your entire vertebral column. Release and repeat.

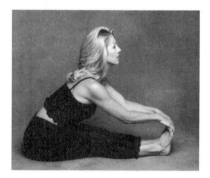

Back Extension, Level I—Cobra. Lie facedown with your hands directly under your shoulders, palms facing down, fingers pointed forward. Exhale and tighten your buttocks muscles as you lift your head, shoulders and chest off the floor, dropping your hips and lengthening forward; don't use your arm muscles to push yourself up. Focus on your buttocks instead. Squeeze your buttock muscles and lengthen your spine. Picture a snake. Hold for 3 deep breaths, then lower to starting position.

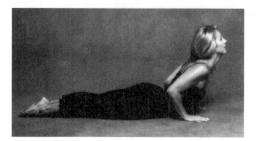

Exercise: Burn Back the Clock!

Back Extension, Level II—Superman. Lie on your belly with your arms and legs extended and your feet about 6 inches apart. Squeeze your buttocks as you slowly raise your head, your arms and your legs an inch or two off the floor. Slowly circle your arms out to your sides and then behind you, palms facing up. Look down at the floor to keep your neck in alignment and anchor your hips to the floor. Concentrate on using proper form—don't overarch your back. Hold for 5 to 10 seconds, then release. Repeat 2 times.

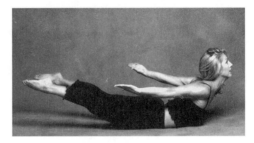

Side Bend (Lateral Flexion). Kneel on the floor with your feet tucked under your bottom. With your arms extended straight up overhead, clasp your hands and stretch upward. Feel the stretch through your waist. Maintaining the stretch, bend your body to the right and take three deep breaths. Return to an upright position, then bend to the left. Take 3 deep breaths. Repeat.

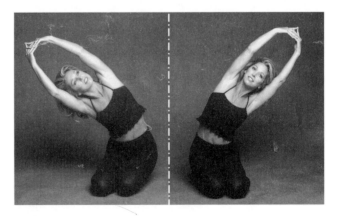

Back Relaxer. Lying down with a pillow underneath your neck and shoulders, let your upper body totally relax into the floor. Gently bring your knees in toward your chest while holding the backs of your legs—your hamstrings. Hold this position for about 30 seconds or as long as it feels good for you. Then gently rock knees slowly to one side, then to the other.

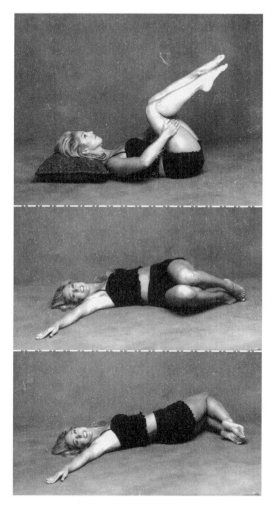

HIP OPENERS

Women's hips are different from men's. Our hip socket is called a Q socket, and unlike men, the line from knee to hip isn't straight; our femurs, or upper leg bones, fit into the hip socket at an angle. For this reason, women tend to experience more hip problems as they grow older.

Hip problems can make walking difficult and lead to back pain and other injuries. You need to keep those hips loose and pliable, particularly as you age. Creaky joints aren't a fact of life—they can be prevented!

Here are three soothing stretches that zero in on those tight, achy hips to promote healthier joints and prevent stiffness and pain. I try to do one or two every day, either first thing in the morning, right before bed, or while watching TV. Start by taking some deep breaths or marching in place (for about 60 seconds) to get the blood flowing and loosen up your muscles. With each exercise you should feel a nice stretch in your hip area, but you shouldn't experience any pain. On a scale of 1 (no stretch whatsoever) to 10 (maximum stretch), aim for a 5 or a 6. Breathe into each stretch and relax your body—don't fight it!

Standing Hip Opener. Stand on your left foot and place your right ankle on your left thigh, right knee bent out to the side. Keeping your knees bent, bend at the hips slightly and push your buttocks back, placing both hands on leg. You can use a chair or wall for balance. Hold for 15 to 30 seconds. Switch sides and repeat.

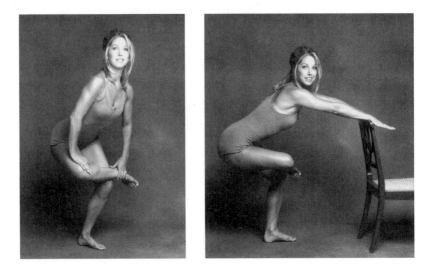

Hip Opener (Advanced). As in the Standing Hip Opener, place your right ankle on your left thigh, right knee bent out to the side. Bend at the hips slightly and push your buttocks back, this time reaching down to the floor. Hold for 15 to 30 seconds. Switch sides and repeat.

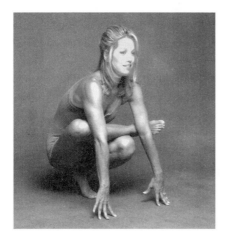

Hip Stretch (Advanced). Sit on the floor with your right leg stretched behind you and your left leg folded in front of you. Place both hands on the floor for balance. Keep your hips down as you lift your chest and let your whole spine lengthen. Hold for 10 seconds. Switch sides and repeat.
Variation: Lower your head and chest to the floor and stretch your arms out to the sides.

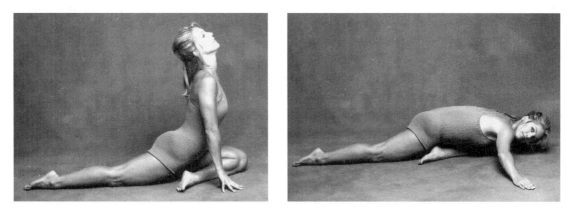

Outer Hip Reliever. Lie on your back with your knees bent and cross your right ankle over your left thigh. Raise your left foot off the floor and place both hands behind your left thigh for support (your left knee should point directly up toward the ceiling). For a deeper stretch, gently pull your left thigh toward you as you use your right elbow to press your right thigh very gently. Hold for 15 to 30 seconds. Switch sides and repeat.

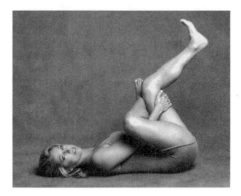

ANTI-GRAVITY EXERCISES

There are five areas of the body that tend to sag with age: your bust, the backs of your upper arms, your waistline, your buns, and the area right above your knees. These are definitely the over-40 problem spots! You can do my targeted toning exercises to supplement your regular anti-aging routine and transform the shape of your body. Remember the rule: If your muscles are toned and taut, nothing can droop or sag!

For each of the five target body parts, I've provided three targeted, anti-gravity toning moves. With these exercises, you'll be creating resistance yourself by contracting or squeezing your target muscle during the move. Remember: Toning exercises are the key to changing the shape of your body. Do these moves 2 to 3 times per week for firmer muscles in as little as three weeks. If you want to use light dumbbells for some of these exercises, go ahead—the more tension on the muscle, the better the results.

On the following pages you'll also find one "invisible" tightening and toning exercise for each body part; these 60-second insta-toners can be done anytime, anywhere. Try to do them at least once a day! For best results, be sure to stretch each area after you work it.

BEAUTIFUL BUST

Strong chest muscles are essential for statuesque posture and to make saggy breasts look more firm and lifted. For a younger, more feminine figure—regardless of your age—do these chest exercises 2 to 3 times a week. For best results, be sure to keep your abdominals tight and don't arch your lower back.

Cleavage Enhancer. Have one foot in front of the other for balance and stability. Lean forward slightly. While holding your weights with wrists straight, begin with arms wide and rounded, elbows slightly bent. Then, with control, pull your arms toward one another, crossing the arms in front. Do 2 sets of 8 to 12 repetitions, alternating.
Benefits: Firms and strengthens your pectorals (chest).

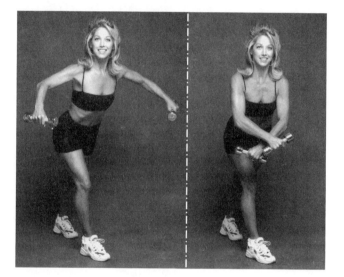

Bust Line Lift. Stand with your feet together, knees bent and back nice and straight. Place your arms in front, shoulder level with palms facing each other. Quickly, with a pulsing motion, press palms in and apart without actually touching hands together. Do 20 to 25 tiny contractions, pulsing inward.
Benefits: Will give you a natural breast lift, toning the chest muscles.

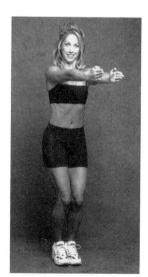

Exercise: Burn Back the Clock!

Bust Booster. Begin in a bent-knee push-up position with your hands spread as wide as possible. Focus on using your chest muscles as you do a push-up, bending your arms to lower your chest toward the floor. Do 2 sets of 8 to 12 reps.
Benefits: Strengthens and firms your entire chest muscle.

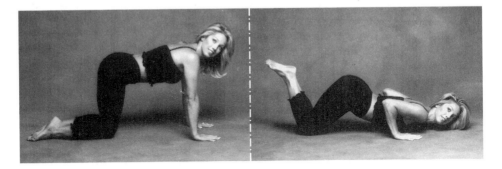

60-Second Chest Developer. Kneel and bring the heels of your palms together in front of your chest (or place your hands in prayer position). Press your hands together for 10 seconds. Feel your chest muscles working. Relax for 5 seconds. Repeat the sequence 3 to 4 times.
Benefits: Firms and tones your chest.

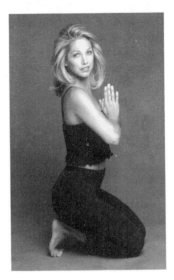

Chest Stretch. Clasp your fingers behind your neck. Pull your elbows back as far as you can. Hold for 10 seconds. Keeping your fingers clasped, try to bring your elbows together in front of you. Hold for 5 seconds. Release your hands and relax for 5 seconds. Repeat the sequence 3 times.

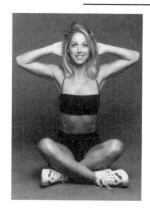

AWESOME ARMS

Your biceps (the front of your arms) get a workout every time you open a car door or lift a bag of groceries, but your triceps (the back of your arms) are rarely called to action in everyday life. Weak triceps muscles (and excess fat, of course) translate to that dreaded upper arm jiggle that's difficult to hide, especially in the summer. Here are some excellent exercises to help you banish those bat wings once and for all!

Arm Series. Stand with your feet together and knees bent for balance. Your arms will extend all the way out to the side from your body. Make two fists and twist the wrists down, then open the hands, palms facing up, and finish by lifting the arms up close to your ears, palms facing each other. Return to standing position and repeat these three moves 10 times for firmer arms.

Benefits: For firmer, sexier-looking arms.

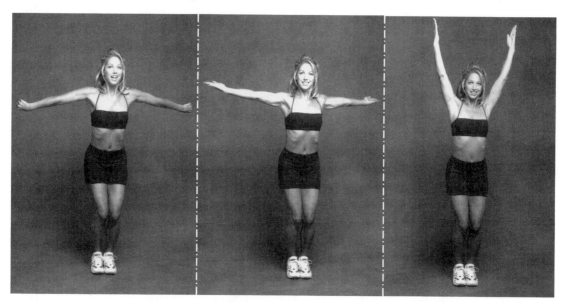

Elbow Strikes. Lunge from side to side with elbow extended, hands in fists with palms facing down. Use momentum and your hips with the lunging motion. Keep your arms and shoulder muscles strong while executing this strike. Do 15 sets using both elbows.
Benefits: Dodge the aging process by toning your upper body.

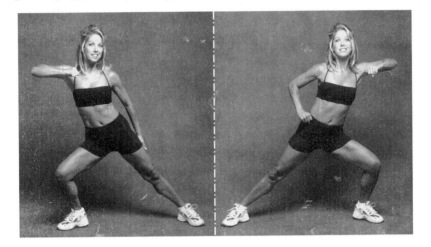

Triceps Toner. In a seated or standing position with your abdominals tight and back straight, hold a weight in your right hand and raise your right arm so that your hand is directly over your right shoulder. Slowly bend your elbow and lower the weight behind your head, as shown, keeping your elbow as close to your head as possible. Squeeze the back of your arm as you raise your hand back over your head to the starting position. Do 2 sets of 8 to 12 reps, then switch arms and repeat.
Benefits: Strengthens and tones your triceps—no more sag!

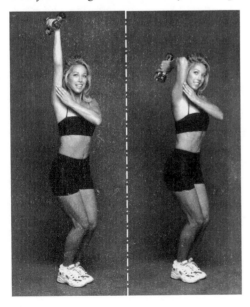 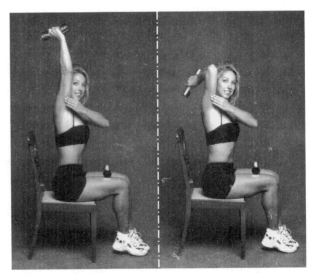

Double Arm Row. Begin with your feet together, knees bent and lean slightly forward. Hold your weights with your palms facing in. With a slow movement, pull the weights back at a diagonal angle using your upper back, shoulders and biceps. Let your shoulders relax, then squeeze your shoulder blades together at the last second for extra-strength work in the back. Do 2 sets of 8 to 12 repetitions.

Benefits: Fight back against gravity with this great exercise to help you firm up.

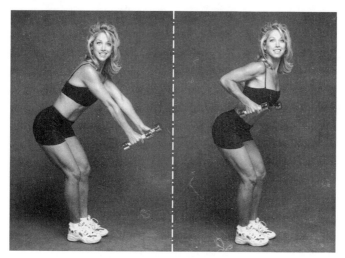

60-Second Triceps Tightener. Stand with your feet together. Extend your arms straight behind you, elbows close in to your body, palms facing the ceiling. Focus on squeezing the back of your arms as you lift your palms up toward the ceiling. Hold for 1 to 2 seconds, then release briefly. Repeat for a total of 1 minute.

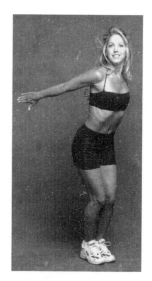

Neck and Shoulder Stretch (Head Tilt). Relax in a comfortable seated position. Right arm rests by your side. Your left fingertips gently tilt and pull your head sideways or toward your shoulder. Do other side. Then, with both hands, gently pull your head forward away from your body. Hold each position for 15 seconds.

Benefits: Releases stress and tension from the neck and shoulders.

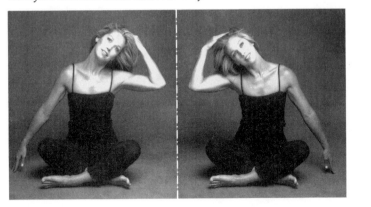 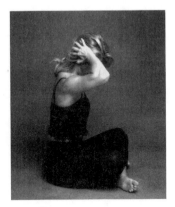

AMAZING ABS

Soft, mushy abdominal muscles not only look terrible in a bathing suit, but can contribute to back pain and poor posture. My guess is that every one of you could stand to do some extra work on your tummy—most people could! The exercises below target your four main abdominal muscles (the rectus abdominis, the transversus and the inner and outer obliques) to help you achieve a firmer, tighter belly. If you have weak abdominals, you may find these moves especially challenging at first, but they should get more doable as you develop your middle muscles. Remember: If you really want to see the effects of these toning exercises, you'll need to get rid of some of the overlying fat through healthy eating and aerobic activity.

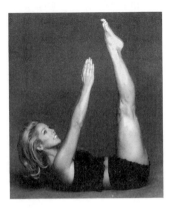

Ab Reach. Lying on your back, lift your legs into the air, forming the letter L with your upper and lower body. Your arms will begin by your side. Then, with abdominal strength, lift up, reaching your hands to your feet. Make sure your legs stay still and your lower back is pressed into the floor to really isolate those ab muscles. Try 20 of these, or as many as you can do.

Benefits: A great toner for the upper and lower abdominal region. Also, this is a good way for building a tall spine and good posture.

Trunk Stabilizer. Begin on your back with both knees bent and arms overhead. Using the muscles in your torso, bring your left knee in toward your chest, at the same time reaching your right arm to your leg. Switch sides and repeat 20 times.

Benefits: You'll feel this working the rectus abdominis (the front part of your abs) and the obliques (the sides of your waist). Super exercise to target your entire middle section.

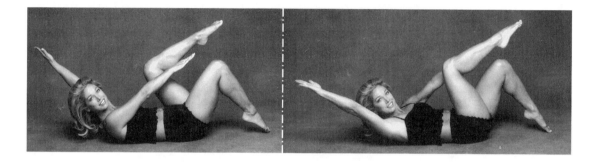

Waistline Trimmer. Lie on your back with your knees bent and feet flat on the floor and place your hands behind your head for support. Contract your abdominals and press the small of your back into the floor as you lift your head and shoulders about 6 inches from the floor. Twist slightly to the side, reaching your elbows to the outside of your right thigh. Hold and pulse (lift up and down slightly) for 5 to 10 seconds, trying to keep your shoulders off the floor. Relax and repeat to the other side for one more set. Do 2 sets of 8 to 12 reps on each side.

Benefits: Tightens and tones your oblique muscles to create waistline contour.

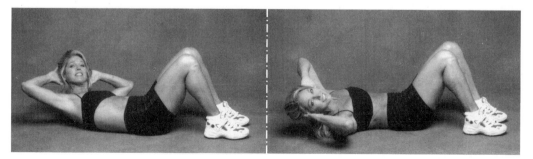

Tummy Tuck. Balancing on your tailbone and seat, let your hands hold you up. Legs will extend in front, creating a V with the body. Pull knees into the chest, crossing at the ankles. Alternate the crossing of the ankles 8 to 12 times.

Variation: An exercise to target the "love handle" or oblique area—keep the knees together and twist at the waist, knees pulling in alternating shoulders, also done 8 to 12 times. This is a challenging move.

Benefits: This will isolate the upper and lower abdominal area and the entire waistline, with the variation included.

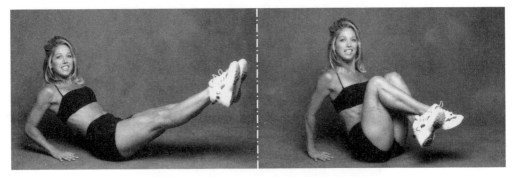

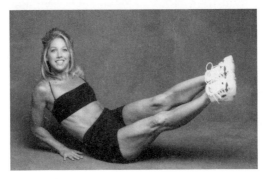

60-Second Ab Firmer. Exhale as you "tuck in" your tummy and contract the abdominal muscles as hard as you can. Hold for 3 to 5 seconds, then inhale as you release. Repeat contracting and relaxing for 1 minute. I do this belly buster practically everywhere, including cars and airplanes!

Abdominal Stretch. Lie on your back with your arms stretched over-head. Stretch your hands away from your toes to lengthen your abdominal region. Hold for 15 to 30 seconds. Try a rolled towel or exercise ball under your back for an extra stretch to create more length through the abdominals.

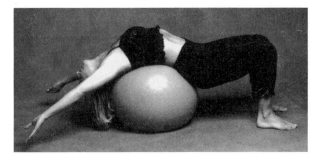

Tips for Building Amazing Abs

- During floor exercises, keep your lower back pressed firmly to the floor throughout the movement.

- To prevent unnecessary strain on your neck and upper back, don't pull on the back of your head to lift yourself—use your abs instead.

- Exhale as you contract or "crunch" and inhale as you release; it may seem awkward, but it's key to a flat, firm tummy.

- Slower is better to make sure you're using your muscles, not momentum.

BETTER BUNS

Most of us spend way too much time sitting in front of our TVs and computers or in our cars. Since your buttock muscles go to work with every step you take, it's no wonder our butts are getting soft and droopy! Strong gluteals, or buttock muscles, will give your derriere a wonderful shape. As you do these exercises, focus on contracting or squeezing your buttock muscles. Remember: If you don't squeeze it, no one else will!

Tush Tightener. Kneel on the floor on all fours, hands directly beneath your shoulders, knees beneath your hips. Keeping your back flat, abs tight and hips square to the floor, raise your right leg out, keeping it bent at a 90-degree angle, until your thigh is parallel to the floor. Slowly lower your knee back down to relax, and then back up again, squeezing your buttocks. Continue until you've completed 2 sets of 8 to 12, then switch legs. To add resistance, use an ankle weight.
Benefits: Tones and firms your buttocks (gluteus maximus).

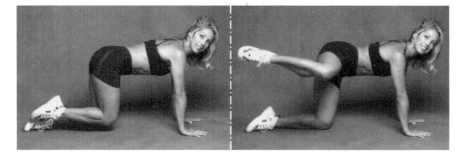

Tush Toner. You'll want to start this in a push-up position on the palms of your hands and the balls of you feet—also known as Plank Position. Abs are in. Back stays straight. Squeeze your buttocks. Lift one foot 6 to 8 inches off the floor and hold for 5 seconds. Return to Plank and repeat. Do 2 more sets.
Benefits: Anti-aging and anti-gravity for the rear end. Keep it up and firm! Also a great trunk stabilizer.

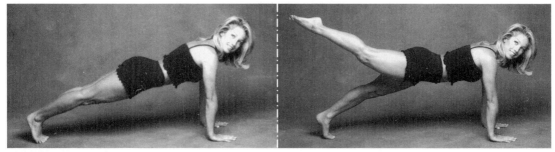

Buns Blaster. Stand with one foot in front of the other and arms extended out to the sides. Bend front knee and point your back foot toward the floor so you're balancing on your front leg. Bend the knee of your standing leg to lower yourself down slightly, squeezing your buttocks muscles. Now, lift and lower the back leg 8 to 12 times. Relax and repeat with the other leg. (Don't do these if you have bad knees.) If you're a beginner, hold on to a wall or chair for balance.
Benefits: Isolates and strengthens your buttocks (gluteals); improves balance.

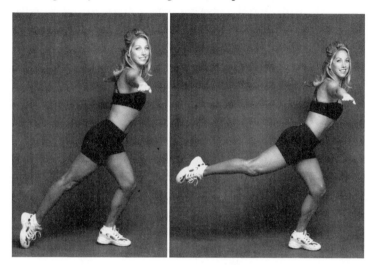

60-Second Butt Blaster. A perfect exercise, whether you're waiting in line at the store or in a chair at your doctor's office (unless you're wearing tight jeans)! Squeeze your buttocks together for five seconds, then release. (This is equal to one squat). Continue squeezing and releasing for 1 minute.

Best Buns Stretch. Sit with your legs crossed in front of you and reach your arms in front with both hands. Feel the stretch. Now gently walk your fingertips to the side over one knee and then the other. You should feel the stretch in your right buttock cheek and then the left buttock cheek. Hold for 10 to 15 seconds in each direction.

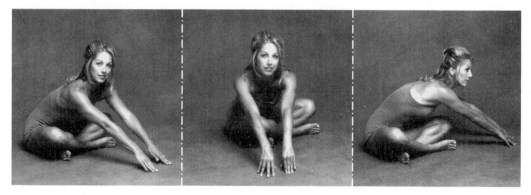

LOVELY LEGS

I know women who rarely miss a day of jogging, yet the area just above their knees still look flabby. Here are some easy exercises to tighten and tone the muscles in this spot. Not only will these moves help you achieve sexy Tina Turner legs, they can help prepare you for sports like tennis and skiing. They're perfect for anyone with bad knees!

Quads Sculptor. Sit on the floor with your knees bent, feet on the floor. To make it easier, lean back on your elbows, fingers facing forward. Slowly extend one leg straight in front of you, foot flexed, and tighten the top of your thigh. Lift leg one foot off the floor, then lower. Do 8 to 12 reps with each leg.
Variation: For a more advanced exercise, sit up straight and bend one knee. Hold the bent knee.
Benefits: Strengthens and tones your quadriceps (front of your thighs).

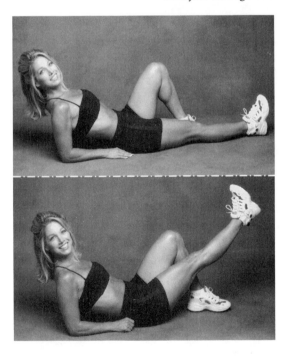

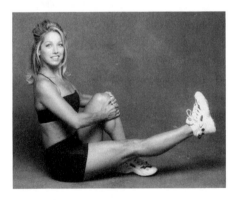

Inner Thigh Shaper. Repeat the Quads Sculptor with toes turned out to the side to work the inner thighs. Do 1 to 2 sets of 8 to 12 reps with each leg.
Benefits: Firms the inner part of your thighs, especially around the inner part of your kneecap.

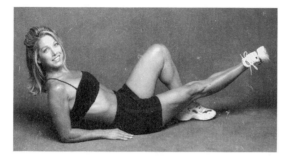

Leg Swing. Lie on your side, resting your head on a pillow, left arm extended overhead. Right arm is bent, resting in front of your chest, supporting your upper body, fingertips touching the floor. Hips are stacked one on top of the other. Your right top leg swings forward, creating an L with your legs, then swing back with perfect control in the opposite direction. Continue this fluid forward-and-back motion 8 to 10 times, keeping the pelvis in neutral positon. Only the legs will be moving. Your middle and upper body should stay still. Squeeze the buttocks so that your back does not over-arch. Relax and switch sides.
Benefits: Excellent toning for the front and back of the thighs. Also will strengthen your hips and the core of your body (the torso area).

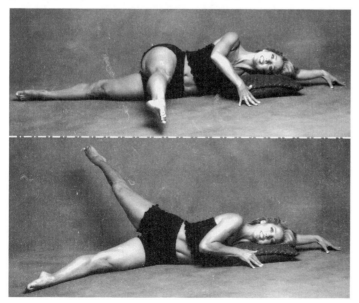

Exercise: Burn Back the Clock!

Inner Thigh Squeeze. Stand with feet about shoulder-width apart. Keep knees bent. Place the palms of your hands directly above the knees on the inner thigh area. Use your upper body for resistance and to create a degree of difficulty with this move at the same time your knees are pushing together. Do 10 to 20 repetitions of the in-and-out movement. *Benefits: Targets the inner thighs, shaping and firming, just like a weight machine, but you're using your own body for resistance, which adds upper body toning—chest, shoulders, biceps and triceps.*

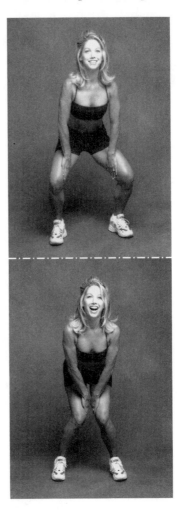

Leg Series. First, to target the inner thighs, begin with your feet shoulder-width apart, a soft bend in your knees for balance. Lift one leg up 6 inches off the floor with the instep of your foot facing up to the ceiling, squeezing and focusing on your inner thigh. Repeat on other side. Next, to target the outer thighs, alternate a side, and lift toes barely off the floor. For balance, lean a little in the opposite direction of the leg you are lifting. Finally, lean slightly forward, alternating lifts behind you—squeeze your glut (your rear) and the hamstring (back of your leg). Do 6 to 8 sets for both legs for each of these three exercises.

Variation: I'm using an exercise band wrapped around my ankles for greater resistance. If you don't have one, don't worry, you can do the same exercises with ankle weights. Or just use your own body weight for resistance, especially if you're just starting out.

Benefits: Great for those trouble spots—hips, thighs and buns. Reverse the aging process with these three exercises.

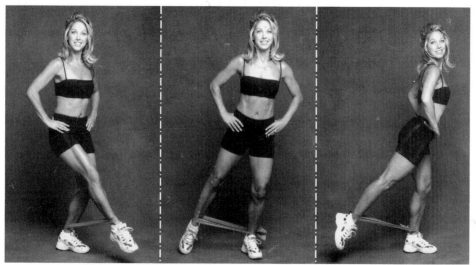

60-Second Quads Firmer. You can do this thigh toner whenever you're sitting. Extend one leg, foot flexed, up as high as possible. Hold for 5 to 10 seconds. Lower. Repeat for a total of 1 minute.

Benefits: Strengthens the muscles surrounding your knees, and promotes circulation.

Quad Stretch. Stand with your feet together and hold on to a wall or a chair for balance. Bend your right knee behind you and hold your foot with your right hand. Gently pull your heel toward your buttocks and feel the stretch in the front of your thigh. Hold for 15 to 30 seconds. Switch legs and repeat.

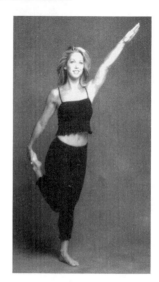

Exercise: Burn Back the Clock!

YOUR 28-DAY CHALLENGE

Now that you know how to exercise your way to a younger, healthier, more energetic body, it's time to get moving! Below, you'll find your basic workout goals for the next four weeks and beyond. If you're a regular exerciser (you've been working out consistently for the past six months), you can jump right into the "Ultimate Weekly Challenge." But if you're a beginner, I want you to start with the "Beginner Challenge," which allows you to build strength and endurance gradually. Don't forget: If you overdo it in the beginning, you'll only get sore, which can really zap your motivation. It's better to take it slowly and focus on your ultimate goal—exercising for a *lifetime.*

BEGINNER CHALLENGE:

Week 1: Cardio: 10 minutes, 3 to 4 times per week
Strength: 30 minutes, 1 time per week
Flexibility/Balance: 5 to 10 minutes, 2 times per week

Week 2: Cardio: 15 minutes, 3 to 4 times per week
Strength: 30 minutes, 1 to 2 times per week
Flexibility/Balance: 5 to 10 minutes, 3 times per week

Week 3: Cardio: 20 minutes, 3 to 4 times per week
Strength: 30 minutes, 2 times per week
Flexibility/Balance: 5 to 10 minutes, 4 times per week

Week 4: Cardio: 25 minutes, 3 to 4 times per week
Strength: 30 minutes, 2 to 3 times per week
Flexibility/Balance: 5 to 10 minutes, 5 times per week

Week 5: Progress to the Ultimate Challenge

ULTIMATE WEEKLY CHALLENGE:

Cardio: 30 minutes, 3 to 4 times per week
Strength: 30 minutes, 2 to 3 times per week
Flexibility/Balance: 5 to 10 minutes, 6 times per week

Remember: The Ultimate Challenge is the minimum amount of exercise needed to keep your heart, bones and joints healthy, your reflexes sharp and your metabolism revved. As you get in better shape, you may want to adjust your goals so your body stays challenged—say, by adding 5 or 10 minutes to your cardio workouts or doing an extra flexibility/balance workout.

Use the Workout Log found on pages 110–12 to keep track of your progress. If you've met all of your goals at the end of 28 days, give yourself a healthy reward such as a brand-new pair of workout shoes or an extra hour of sleep. You deserve it!

PROGRESS REPORT

Before starting my Stop the Clock program, take these simple tests to assess your aerobic capacity, strength, flexibility and balance. Repeat the tests at the end of four weeks to see how far you have come.

There's one thing that I want to clarify. When we talk about losing weight, we're really talking about losing excess body fat. With a combination of exercise and healthy, low-fat eating, you can shed that extra flab and improve the shape of your body. But in this program, you'll be strength-training, which means that as you lose fat you'll be *adding* muscle to speed up your metabolism and guard your body against osteoporosis and other by-products of aging. Since muscle weighs more than fat, the bathroom scale may not be an accurate monitor of your success. Rather than getting obsessed with the numbers, concentrate on how your body looks and feels—you'll notice the difference when your dress size goes down from a 14 to a 10, or when you make it up the stairs without huffing and puffing.

The most accurate way to evaluate your progress is to get your body fat measured. Many health clubs offer skin-fold or electronic imaging tests; these tests may not be 100 percent accurate, but they can give you an idea of how you're doing in terms of fat loss. After a few weeks of exercise and good eating habits, you can get retested to see roughly how much fat you've managed to shed. Another good way to monitor your progress is to use a tape measure or check your clothes. Have you lost inches around your thighs and belly? Are your pants looser? Do your hips, thighs and tummy feel firmer and less jiggly? Remember, even if you've lost only a pound or two on the scale, you've added muscle and gotten rid of fat, which is your ultimate goal.

AEROBIC CAPACITY
How far can you walk in five minutes?

DAY 1: _____

DAY 28: _____

STRENGTH
The 1-Minute Push-up Test
- Rest your weight on your hands and knees, hands shoulder-width apart, lower legs bent up at a 90-degree angle. (Crossing your ankles will increase your stability.)
- Your body should form a straight line from head to knees.
- Bend your elbows, lowering your body until your chest all but touches the floor; do not break the line of your body by letting your waist bend or your stomach droop.

Exercise: Burn Back the Clock!

Workout Log

One of the best ways to measure your success and stay motivated is to record your workouts. I've provided space for you to write down the date and duration of each exercise session as well as details on what you did and how it felt. Before filling it in, I recommend making copies of this weekly log to use for the next four weeks and after the program is over. If you miss a workout, be sure to note the reasons why you couldn't get to it. At the end of each week, pat yourself on the back for your accomplishments. If you don't achieve your goals, consider why. By recognizing your exercise obstacles, you'll prevent them from getting in your way again.

Week 1
CARDIO: 30 minutes, 3 to 4 times a week
Workout 1
Date _____   Activity _____   Duration _____
Notes _____

_____

_____

Workout 2
Date _____   Activity _____   Duration _____
Notes _____

_____

_____

Workout 3
Date _____   Activity _____   Duration _____
Notes _____

_____

_____

Workout 4
Date _____   Activity _____   Duration _____
Notes _____

_____

_____

STRENGTH TRAINING: 20–30 minutes, 2 or 3 times per week

Workout 1

Date _____ Routine _____ Duration _____

Notes _____

_____

_____

Workout 2

Date _____ Routine _____ Duration _____

Notes _____

_____

_____

Workout 3

Date _____ Routine _____ Duration _____

Notes _____

_____

_____

FLEXIBILITY/BALANCE: 5–10 minutes, 6 times per week

Workout 1

Date _____ Activity _____ Duration _____

Notes _____

_____

_____

Workout 2

Date _____ Activity _____ Duration _____

Notes _____

_____

_____

Workout 3

Date _____   Activity _____   Duration _____

Notes _____

_____

_____

Workout 4

Date _____   Activity _____   Duration _____

Notes _____

_____

_____

Workout 5

Date _____   Activity _____   Duration _____

Notes _____

_____

_____

Workout 6

Date _____   Activity _____   Duration _____

Notes _____

_____

_____

- Raise yourself up to the starting position, extending your arms fully.
- See how many push-ups you can do in 1 minute.

Your Results

DAY 1: _____

DAY 28: _____

The 1-Minute Crunch Test

- Place a strip of tape on the floor.
- Lie on your back with your knees bent directly over the piece of tape, your feet flat on the floor.

- Press your shoulders against the floor and extend your arms along your sides. Your fingertips should be about 3 inches from the tape. Place your palms flat on the floor.
- Lift your head and shoulders off the floor in a partial sit-up or crunch, coming up only as far as necessary for your fingers to touch the tape.
- Release.
- Do as many of these crunches as you can in 1 minute, counting each time your fingers touch the tape. Be sure that your shoulders touch the floor after each crunch.
- If you can do more than 40 of these in 1 minute, WOW!

Your Results
DAY 1: _____
DAY 28: _____

FLEXIBILITY
The Sit-and-Reach Test
- Place a strip of tape on the floor.
- Place a yardstick perpendicular to the tape at the 14-inch mark, with the 1-inch mark toward your body.
- Sit on the floor and extend your legs straight in front of you, straddling the yardstick.
- Place your heels on the floor about 5 inches apart, so that they just touch the near edge of the tape.
- Keeping your legs straight, reach forward, with your hands side by side (do not lead with one hand).
- Touch the yardstick as far away as you can.
- Reach slowly and hold; do not bounce. See how close you can come to touching your toes.
- Record how far you stretch.

Your Results
DAY 1: _____
DAY 28: _____

BALANCE
The One-Legged Test
- Stand on your right leg.
- Place your hands on your hips.
- Raise your left foot in front of you, about 6 inches off the floor.

- Keep your balance as long as you can without letting your left foot touch the floor (focusing your gaze several inches in front of you will help).
- Count how many seconds go by before you lose your balance.

Your Results
DAY 1: _____
DAY 28: _____

STAYING MOTIVATED

Okay, that's it, you're finally convinced—you need to start exercising TODAY. I hate being the bearer of bad news, but starting a fitness program is the easy part. Keeping it going is a whole other matter. As my friend George Allen, the famous former coach of the Washington Redskins, says, a workout is 25 percent perspiration and 75 percent determination. So it's time to get determined!

While we all dream of the magic pill that will help us regain our youth and shed pounds without lifting a finger, it simply doesn't exist. There will never be a drug that strengthens our hearts, firms our muscles and helps us lose weight permanently. To get lasting health benefits, you need to make exercise a part of your life *forever*. Unfortunately, most new exercisers abandon their workout regimens within six months of starting them. Here are some tips to make sure that you aren't one of them!

Set clear goals. As I said earlier, for the next four weeks I'll be helping you form specific exercise goals. But once this program is over, you should continue setting new daily and weekly goals (i.e., how many minutes of cardio you'll do today or how many times you'll work out this week). Make each exercise session a priority—no skipping. You're not the only one who loses when you miss a workout—your family loses, too!

Think beyond weight loss. Yes, exercise can help you keep your waistline in check, but don't do it just to drop that extra weight. If you're going to stick with it, you need to enjoy the process. Try focusing on how wonderful your body feels when it is strong and more limber. Think about your healthy heart. Picture yourself in that great new sexy dress. Visualize your grandson's college graduation. Talk about incentive!

Schedule your workouts. Plan your workouts for a specific time each day—even write them down on your calendar—and treat them like an important doctor's appointment that you just can't miss.

Exercise Angels

If you have trouble staying motivated, try one of these inspiring strategies:
Join a walking club
Get a dog—or borrow your neighbor's
Exercise with someone younger
Buy a new workout outfit or exercise video
Plan an active vacation

Keep an activity log. Writing down the specifics of each exercise session, including how you felt afterward, will help you track your progress and keep you motivated. (You'll find a space to do this starting on page 110!)

Make exercise convenient. I'm all for investing in home equipment like a treadmill or a stationary bike. It's much easier to grab 15 minutes on the bike while the chicken is defrosting than to drive to the gym!

Don't "settle" on a workout. If you dislike the stationary bike and hate the stair climber, keep trying new machines or workouts until you find one you can live with or maybe even enjoy. Remember: An aerobic workout doesn't have to feel like work—and it doesn't have to take place under a roof. Tennis, volleyball, soccer, in-line skating, cross-country skiing and snowshoeing can all be great cardio workouts.

Vary your activities. We all love routines, but they can make our workouts boring and impede our progress. Plus it's amazing how time whizzes by when you try a new sport or activity. Pick up a new workout video, try a new dance class or sign up for tennis lessons for a fun change.

Keep moving! Even on super-busy days, be sure to incorporate 5 to 10 minutes of movement. Better yet, try 5 to 10 minutes three times a day. It's easier than you think, and it only takes a little bit of exercise to keep your body in the mood and craving more.

Exercise Evils

Five energy drains to avoid:
Hanging out with non-fitness friends
Watching TV
Heavy lunches
Junk food
Alcoholic beverages

Exercise: Burn Back the Clock!

Challenge yourself. Don't always stick to what feels comfortable and "easy"; every once in a while, push yourself to the edge. If you've never jogged more than two miles, try jogging two and a half miles. Increase the incline on the treadmill or go for your fastest-ever time. Prove to yourself that you can do it! As your fitness level increases, so will your motivation to continue.

Bottom line: No one can talk you into exercising—not even me. You have to want to make these changes for YOU. If you feel your determination faltering, keep reminding yourself of all the wonderful benefits—a svelte waistline, better skin, less stress and more confidence, to name just a few. Then, consider the possible what-ifs of *not* exercising: insulin injections starting in your 40s, a triple bypass operation in your 50s, a stroke in your 60s, and a fractured hip or debilitating arthritis in your 70s. If those aren't reasons to keep moving, I don't know what is!

Get moving or get left behind!

Ask Denise

Starting and maintaining a regular exercise program takes hard work and dedication. And if you're like me, anything new requires thought and planning, with loads of new questions to be answered. Learning as much as possible before beginning can help boost your confidence and prevent potential pitfalls. Here are answers to some common questions.

Q. Should I join a gym?
A. If you can afford it and it helps keep you motivated, a gym membership is a great idea. You'll have access to a wide variety of equipment and professional advice. Many people also enjoy the social aspect of going to the gym. It serves as an opportunity to get out of the house and interact with other people, and it creates a sense of belonging. Concerned you won't fit in? These days gyms aren't just for burly bodybuilders: According to the International Health and Racquet Sports Association, more than half (53 percent) of all club members are women, and almost 25 percent are over age 35. If you're just not a gym person, don't worry: You can get all the benefits of my anti-aging exercise program at home. You may need to invest in a few minor pieces of equipment, like dumbbells or exercise videos. But those items can be purchased quite inexpensively.

Q. When is the best time to exercise?
A. Whenever you're most likely to do it. Personally, I like working out in the morning. It helps wake me up, puts me in a good mood and gets my metabolism revved right away. And then it's not hanging over my

head for the rest of the day! By exercising first thing, I also eliminate the chances of running out of time later. But for you night owls, the evening is just as effective.

Q. What if I have a bad back?

A. For cardio, stick with non-impact workouts like swimming or aqua aerobics. If you don't have access to a pool, the stair climber or the elliptical machine at your gym are your safest bets. Whatever happens, don't skip your crunches (page 54) or your single-leg exercises (pages 80–81). Increasing your abdominal and lower back strength is the best way to prevent back pain as well as future back problems! If you have severe or chronic pain, be sure to consult your physician or physical therapist before beginning any new exercises.

Q. What's the best workout for burning fat?

A. Interval training, alternating bursts of high-intensity exercise ("work") with lower-intensity exercise ("recovery"). Research shows that this type of high/low-intensity training burns fat more effectively than a continuous steady-state workout. Why? Pushing your heart to the maximum allows you to burn more calories; by allowing yourself to catch your breath and recover, you're able to sustain this elevated pace for longer. Interval training translates to many different workouts, including walking, cycling and swimming. Warning: Interval training isn't for everyone. You need to be in fairly good shape, and you shouldn't try it if you have a history of heart problems. When in doubt, talk to your doctor.

Q. My weight falls in the normal range for my height, but my doctor still suggests that I lose 5 or 10 pounds. Is this really necessary?

A. Sounds like another question for your doctor. What I can tell you is this: Every person and physique is different. Some women with big frames can be healthy carrying a little extra weight. Others with small bones may be better off with less. Since muscle weighs more than fat, getting a body fat measuement may be a more accurate way to gauge your health than stepping on a scale. Anywhere between 20 and 25 percent body fat is considered normal and healthy for most women. I recommend asking your family physician about body fat testing, or head to your local health club.

Q. What if I start to feel pain while exercising? Should I try to work through it?

A. Absolutely not. If you feel pain, stop exercising immediately. If you think it's a muscle strain, apply R.I.C.E.: rest, ice, compression and elevation. Consult your physician if the pain persists more than a day or two or if you think it may be something more serious. And don't return to physical activity without your doctor's okay.

Q. I have skinny legs and a potbelly. Is it possible to lose fat just from my middle?
A. Not really. When you lose body fat through diet and exercise, you lose it from all over your body. That said, you *can* do toning exercises like crunches to tighten that tummy, which will make it appear thinner. And since it's a little easier to lose fat from your abdominal area than other parts of your body, like your thighs and hips, you may find that your belly is the first thing to shrink when you lose flab.

Q. What should I eat before exercising?
A. A pre-exercise meal should be easy to digest and, like any other meal, include a healthy balance of energy-giving carbohydrates, lean protein and fat. For breakfast, try oatmeal, skim milk and a banana. A grilled-chicken salad with light vinaigrette and a 7-grain roll makes a nice lunch. Yogurt and a piece of fruit is a perfect power snack. Whatever you choose, keep it light. If blood is rushing to your stomach to help you digest a large meal, your muscles and joints won't get their due. Otherwise, leave several hours to digest before your workout begins. And don't even think about exercising on an empty stomach. As soon as your tummy starts to grumble, you'll be tempted to cut your workout short.

Q. Do I really need to warm up before a workout?
A. Yes. To avoid injury, it's important to ease your body into a workout with a few minutes of gentle activity—say, a few easy laps before swimming or a brisk walk before jogging. Ideally, your warm-up should include movements that you'll be using in your workout. For instance, a few waist twists and practice swings will help prepare your body for a golf game. It only takes a few extra minutes, and you'll feel better, play better and help protect yourself against painful muscle strains and tears.

Q. Should my warm-up include stretching?
A. Contrary to popular belief, stretching before a workout doesn't reduce your risk of injury—or so the bulk of the research indicates. The latest evidence comes from the University of Sydney, where researchers found that army recruits who stretched before each boot camp workout were just as likely to get hurt as those who didn't. But gentle stretches at the end of your workout *are* important for preventing tight, sore muscles.

Q. I keep hearing about the importance of weight-bearing workouts as we age. What exactly is weight-bearing exercise?

A. Weight-bearing exercise includes everything from strength-training workouts using dumbbells to toning moves like push-ups and sit-ups. It also means any activity that requires lifting your own body weight through space—for example, cardio workouts such as walking, jogging and climbing stairs. (Swimming and the elliptical machine are not weight-bearing workouts). This type of exercise helps strengthen the muscles around your joints and fortify your bones. It's important at any age, but especially as you get older, when muscles get weaker, joints get tight and achy, and bones become more brittle.

Q. The only way I can find time to exercise is by cutting back on sleep. What's more important—sleep or a workout?

A. Both are important, so you need to find another way to make time for exercise. You're the perfect candidate for doing 10-minute workouts throughout the day. Shave 10 minutes off your getting-ready-for-work time, reserve 10 minutes during your lunch or coffee break and squeeze in 10 minutes before dinner, and suddenly you have a full 30 minutes of activity. It's not going to be easy—and it will require changing a habit or two. But it can be done. I've even been known to ride a stationary bike while I'm on a conference call.

So be creative. And remember: strong body, strong mind!

4

Nutrition: Fabulous Foods for Over 40

Whenever I meet a friend or business associate for a meal at a restaurant, they always wait to see what I order.

"Oh, you go first, Denise," they say, peering at me over the menu.

I know from experience they expect me to order the spinach salad with one bean sprout on the side. I love to see their reaction when I pipe up, "I'll have the chicken Parmesan."

Then I let them in on a secret: I adore food. In fact, I *love* food.

I just don't abuse it.

My mom was a terrific cook, and my sisters, brother and I grew up surrounded by the smells of a warm kitchen. All of our family celebrations centered on food: family recipes from my grandmother, special dishes based on what was fresh and in season. Even now, when I get together with my family on vacation, our liveliest debates are based on where to eat dinner!

Of course, I've had to modify my calorie intake over the years to match the natural slowing of my metabolism, but I've never deprived myself of the foods I love. I've just learned to eat smaller portions. Eating more frequent, smaller meals throughout the day actually helps you burn more calories, as it keeps your metabolism revved up and running around the clock. So chances are I'll eat half that chicken Parmesan and take the rest home. Jeff and I usually end up splitting an entrée when we go out. The easiest way to cut calories is to downscale your idea of what a serving is.

I've also learned that eating unhealthy foods can actually accelerate the aging process. A diet high in saturated fat can be the culprit behind many diseases that we are at risk for as we grow older, including heart disease, diabetes, cancer and arthritis. But the reverse is also true: Eating the right foods can actually undo damage done over the years. New research suggests that cell-damaging free radicals—renegade chemicals produced by the body and by bad habits such as smoking and excessive alcohol consumption—can be combated by antioxidants, special substances found in fruits and vegetables, olive oil, black and green tea, fish, and many other sources. Fish oil—which contains healthy omega-3 fatty acids—is a proven anti-aging weapon, as is garlic, which is loaded with antioxidants. Blueberries, the new wonder food, also contain potent antioxidants and, in a study by the Human Nutrition Research Center on Aging, were found to improve short-term memory and sharpen reaction time. Even chocolate contains phenols, antioxidant chemicals that have been shown to reduce heart disease. (Research has shown that *moderate* chocolate eaters—those who eat it once or twice a month—live longer than people who never eat sweets! But take note: This is not license to binge on bonbons every day. I treat myself to a piece of candy every now and then, and savor it because I only get to enjoy it every once in a while.)

I now take a multivitamin, a calcium supplement, and vitamin E and vitamin C every day. I've also cut down on salt (my family has a history of hypertension, which is exacerbated by a high-salt diet) and caffeine. I eat more brown rice now than I used to, and prefer sweet potatoes to white ones. I'm more likely to reach for low-fat yogurt than ice cream, and I'll use honey instead of sugar.

Can we actually slow down the aging process by choosing foods that are right for our over-40 body?

Absolutely!

Whether you've just turned 40 and have a few extra inches around your waist or are a size 4 grandmom, now is the time to reevaluate your eating habits. Did you know that for every pound you lose, you decrease the pressure on your knees by *four pounds?* With a few simple changes, you can help prevent serious health problems (including osteoporosis) and slow the signs of aging on your skin, eyes, teeth and gums. You can also boost your energy, which will make it easier to stick with the exercise programs in Chapter 3 and participate in an active social life.

What follows in these pages is not a diet—although there's a good chance that you will lose weight. I want you to eat . . . but I want you to eat *well*. With the help of two top nutritionists—Edith Howard Hogan, R.D., an American Dietetic Association spokesperson who has specialized in women's nutrition for 25 years, and Leslie Bonci, R.D., director of sports nutrition for the University of Pittsburgh—I've put together a smart, easy-to-follow plan for fortifying your body as you grow older.

Nutrition: Fabulous Foods for Over 40

Throughout this section I'm going to help you determine your nutritional friends and foes. I'll show you ways to prepare quick, healthy meals at home and how to make smart choices at restaurants. (As we get older and our lifestyles change, many of us tend to eat out more.) I'll explain the latest information on vitamins and minerals that keep your engine running like clockwork. You'll learn the science behind bone-saving calcium, the link between fiber and weight loss, and the ultimate age-defying foods.

I've also included some simple recipes that incorporate wonder foods like soy. Now don't moan until you try a few—even my girls like Soy Smoothies. Think what strong bones, healthy hearts and gorgeous complexions they'll have in their 60s!

For many people, figuring out how to eat for maximum health and staying power is a learning process. You may already realize that greasy potato chips make you feel lethargic, or that a heaping bowl of pasta with no protein leaves you only semi-satisfied. If not, the program here will teach you which foods drain your energy and which ones give you a jump start. Not only will smart food choices keep your body healthy and trim for years to come, they'll help you tackle your workouts with gusto.

F.U.E.L.: *FOOD U* NEED FOR *ENERGY* AND *LIFE*

A healthy diet is important at any age, but it's especially crucial now that we're getting older. All those years of eating the wrong foods and dieting have finally caught up with us. Some of the signs are visible: teeth that aren't as strong, hair and skin that feel dry, an expanding waist. Others are less obvious: Our bones are getting weaker, our immune system is suffering and our arteries are lined with fatty plaque.

As you know, food can have a powerful effect on how you look and feel as well as how your body ages. I like to think of my body like a car. The quality of gas that gets put in the tank affects its performance and its longevity. Unfortunately, most of us aren't getting the fuel we need to keep our engines running their best. A study from the University of California at Berkeley shows that about half of all women consume inadequate amounts of essential nutrients ranging from vitamin A to zinc.

I'll admit it: Eating right hasn't always been easy for me either. In my teens and 20s I didn't always watch what I ate. My diet improved dramatically when I got pregnant with my first child, Kelly. I stopped skipping meals and started eating a better balance of foods as well as more fruits and veggies. Now, as I learn more and more about the importance of good nutrition, I'm grateful that I made those changes early on.

If you haven't already, it's time for you to stop committing nutritional no-nos like dieting and filling up on sweets. To help you do that, I'm going to teach you a new way to think about eating. I call it F.U.E.L.—*Food U* Need for *Energy* and *Life*. From now on, the goal is to keep your system fired up with nutrients that will help fend off illness and keep you energized and looking your healthy best.

I'm certainly not against having an ice cream cone or a gooey slice of pizza once in a while. Life would be a bore if we didn't allow ourselves those occasional indulgences! You just don't want to do it all the time. Furthermore, when you're over 40, it's no longer just about weight loss. It's about life expectancy. Your food choices are crucial now, and when you swallow something unhealthy, you're missing an opportunity to fortify yourself with important vitamins and minerals that will keep you in top shape for years to come.

By seeing food as a form of energy and sustenance, it's much easier to eat in a way that will keep your body in top shape. While your midlife taste buds may crave fries and a milk shake (oh, those hormones!), you'll feel and perform better after grilled chicken and a salad. When you're well nourished, it's also easier to maintain a healthy weight because you feel satisfied and won't be as tempted to fill up with empty calories.

Don't forget that *how* you eat is as important as *what* you eat. The best way to keep your body F.U.E.L.ed is by feeding it small amounts throughout the day. Instead of skipping breakfast and sitting down to an old-fashioned meat-and-potatoes dinner that might be fine for a 20-year-old or a marathon runner, you should aim to eat three small, balanced meals and two snacks daily. Your body processes food more efficiently this way, and research from the U.S. Department of Agriculture shows that it may make you less likely to gain weight as you age.

By not letting your body get too hungry, you can also prevent the spikes and dips in blood sugar that cause moodiness, lethargy and overeating. We all know the feeling: It starts with a tiny rumble in your tummy. Soon you have trouble concentrating. You get grouchy and snap at your coworkers or family. Before long you're a heat-seeking missile looking for the fastest source of energy you can get your hands on—often something sugary like a vending machine candy bar, cookies or ice cream. You end up consuming a lot of empty calories for no good reason: You still don't have the energy to exercise, and it isn't long before you find yourself reaching for more, as the insulin rush sparks your appetite.

With F.U.E.L., I feel like I'm always eating. Every once in a while someone will say to me, "Denise, you never *stop*." I'm not really consuming that many calories, since *what* I'm eating—things like fresh fruit, carrot sticks, raisins or a container of yogurt—is usually healthy and low in calories. But you do need to be careful. This program *isn't* a license to overeat. So try to keep tabs on your portion sizes (more about that on page 131), and don't just eat for the sake of eating. Remember: You're eating for energy and vitality. Every bite counts!

Don't get me wrong—food is more than fuel. It is a form of art, a cozy comfort, a symbol of love and a great excuse to get together with friends. So let's put enjoyment back into it! Instead of wolfing down a bagel for breakfast or stuffing in a sandwich at lunch, I want you to slow down and enjoy each and every bite—which you'll be better able to do if you don't let yourself get too hungry.

Even before you take a bite and as you chew, indulge in the smells, the tastes, the textures and the colors of the food you're eating: bright yellow peppers and cherry tomatoes on a bed of baby green lettuce, raspberries and blueberries on vanilla yogurt, a slice of melon with a sprig of fresh mint, a swirl of yogurt in a sweet roasted-pepper soup, brown rice topped with stir-fried snow peas, red peppers, yellow squash and chicken.

A word about soup: Researchers at Pennsylvania State University recently found that starting a meal with a hot, broth-based soup caused diners to consume 100 fewer calories during the meal. Foods with high water content help us feel full on fewer calories. So start a meal with a delicious broth-based soup (forget the creamy chowders), and feel more satisfied with fewer calories!

TAKE OFF THE POUNDS, TAKE OFF THE YEARS

While food is one of life's pleasures, you need to practice moderation in order to stave off extra inches. As I said earlier, it's critical to maintain a healthy weight as you age—and not just so you feel wonderful when you look in the mirror. When you're overweight, even by just 10 or 15 pounds, you're at much higher risk for heart attack, stroke, diabetes and other serious conditions. For every additional pound you carry, you put unnecessary strain on your back and knees, leaving you too uncomfortable and tired to walk up a flight of stairs or play with your children or grandkids.

Despite the fact that so many people struggle with losing weight, there isn't any magic formula for doing it—at least in theory. I'm sure you've heard of the new wonder drug Xenical (orlistat), which supposedly allows you to eat all the fat you want without gaining weight. Beware! This so-called fat blocker is intended only for women who meet the medical criteria for obesity. There are unpleasant side effects (gas, diarrhea, bloating). Plus, patients who took the drug lost only about six pounds more than those who simply followed a healthy diet. There have been no long-term studies on this drug, and the question of fat absorption is still being debated.

Ephedra is another so-called miracle pill. This substance is not considered a drug; rather, it's an herbal dietary supplement that acts as an appetite suppressant. But if combined with caffeine or cold pills, it can also dangerously tax your cardiovascular and nervous systems. Furthermore, it is difficult to know the proper dose, since ephedra is not regulated by the Food and Drug Administration.

To shed excess fat, you need to burn more calories than you consume. It's as simple as that. How many calories you should take in each day depends on factors like your body weight and how much you exercise. To figure out approximately how many calories you need, you can use this simple equation: Multiply your weight by 13 if you exercise (or by 10 if you don't exercise).

According to the equation, if you weigh 140 pounds and work out regularly, you'll need about 1,800 calories per day to maintain your weight. If you're trying to lose weight, you could drop down to 1,600 calories daily—but don't go any lower. Doing so could cause you to feel deprived and actually slow your metabolism. If you're exercising a lot, you may want to increase your intake to 2,000 calories. Since everyone is different, you have to judge by how your clothes fit and how your body feels. Listlessness during your workouts could be a sign that you need a little more fuel.

One of the worst things that you can do if you're trying to trim down is deprive yourself of food. People who try to lose weight this way are almost guaranteed to fail. Even if the scale shows a big change at first, it won't last. Why? Because your body needs fuel to operate. As we discussed in Chapter 3, when you're depriving yourself of food, your brain tells your body to slow down and conserve energy. Your resting metabolic rate drops. So even if you're eating less, your weight will plateau. You *stop* losing weight because you're not burning as many calories. As soon as you return to your regular eating habits, you start gaining again quickly because your body is still in conservation mode. Sound familiar?

Not only is this kind of drastic dieting bad from a long-term weight-loss standpoint, it's harmful for your body. Starving yourself puts stress on all your internal organs. You lose valuable electrolytes, which can be dangerous for your kidneys and can weaken your immune system. When you're not getting enough energy from food, your body starts breaking down muscle to feed itself, leaving your limbs weak and your metabolism sluggish. You are subject to depression and irritability. You don't have enough energy to exercise. And you miss out on vital nutrients necessary to keep yourself strong, healthy and beautiful. You may lose a few pounds in time for your high school reunion, but then you gain it all back and suffer from low self-esteem.

Ditto for the latest fad, high-protein diets. These diets work by simply restricting calories, not by some special combination of foods. The weight that you lose is apt to be regained when you start eating carbohydrates again (which is almost guaranteed to happen). The long-term effects of protein diets haven't been studied, so doctors don't know what will happen to your body down the road. What they *do* know is that eating a lot of red meat, eggs, cheese and other animal products that are high in saturated fat will make it more likely that you suffer a heart attack or stroke. (Does eating steak and sausage instead of bananas and potatoes really sound healthy to you?)

WHY BALANCE IS BETTER

Variety is indeed the spice of life. In fact, it may actually save your life! Research now shows that people who eat a wide variety of foods live longer than those who don't.

Many of these waist-whittling "miracle" diets that eliminate an entire food group, such as protein or carbohydrates, aren't based on sound scientific research that shows how they affect our bodies over the long haul. They may help you lose weight temporarily, but who knows what they're doing to your bones and arteries? Beware: Any diet that excludes an entire food group or any type of fruit or vegetable is likely to fail—and may be setting you up for other health problems down the line.

All food is made up of three essential macronutrients—carbohydrates, protein and fat. For energy, satiety and a healthy body in general, numerous studies show that a balance of carbs (about 50 to 55 percent of your total calories), protein (about 20 to 25 percent of your daily calories) and fat (about 25 percent of your total calories) is the way to go. Here's why.

Carbohydrates

Carbs are your body's chief source of fuel—you need them for energy. There are two basic types: simple and complex. Simple carbohydrates are foods like cookies that contain a lot of empty calories in the form of sugar, corn syrup, molasses or honey; they do little to nourish your body or curb your appetite. Complex carbs are wholesome foods rich in fiber, vitamins and minerals—such as whole grains, fruits, vegetables and beans—that help fill you up and give you a real energy boost.

Protein

As your body's chief building material, protein provides the necessary ingredients for growing and for repairing muscle, blood, skin and other tissue. While you don't want to go overboard—especially on fatty red meats—it's important to consume adequate amounts. (Research shows that protein requirements may actually increase slightly as we get older.) If you choose to cut out meat, eggs or dairy, be sure to get enough protein from plant sources such as beans, soy and nuts.

Fat

Believe it or not, fats also have a place in a healthy diet. Some fat—especially from the unsaturated fats found in sources like nuts, avocados and fish oil—is needed for energy, supple skin and overall good health. Fat is broken down more slowly than protein or carbohydrate, so it helps you feel satisfied and full. It also brings out the flavor in food—and tasty food is always more gratifying. (That's why fat-free cookies are so unsatisfying. Better to have one real cookie than a bag of fake ones!)

Best Sources of Carbs, Protein and Fat

Carbohydrates
Go for the whole-grain breads, high-fiber cereals, fruits, veggies, brown rice, beans, whole-wheat pasta, potatoes
Skip the cookies, muffins, donuts, white bread, sugary fruit juices

Protein
Go for the fish, shellfish, poultry, beans, white chicken or turkey meat, egg whites, soy, lean red meats, lean pork, low-fat milk, low-fat yogurt, low-fat cheese
Skip the bacon, sausage, cold cuts, fatty meats, hot dogs, liver, dark chicken or turkey meat, whole milk

Fat
Go for the avocados, nuts, olives, vegetable oils (olive, canola, safflower, soybean)
Skip the butter, margarine, shortening, cream, anything fried

That said, dietary fat *will* contribute to weight gain and other health problems if you eat too much of it. According to the National Weight Control Registry, a large-scale study of people who have lost weight and kept it off for more than a year, most individuals who succeed at long-term weight loss adhere to low-fat diets. Furthermore, research shows that a diet low in saturated fat is vital for a healthy heart, and it may help protect your body against breast cancer and other diseases. So try to limit your consumption to about 25 percent or less of your daily calories—and watch your intake of unhealthy saturated and trans fats (we'll discuss these in greater detail on page 165).

Different foods contain different combinations of these basic macronutrients. For instance, a container of low-fat yogurt has carbohydrates

The Healthy Eating Pyramid

Which foods?	How much?	What's a serving?
Fruits and vegetables	5 to 8 servings per day	1 medium apple, banana or orange, ¾ cup vegetable or fruit juice, ¾ cup broccoli, carrots or other vegetables, raw or cooked, 1 medium potato, 1 cup raw leafy vegetables
Meat, poultry, fish, beans, eggs and nuts	2 to 3 servings per day	2–3 ounces cooked meat, poultry or fish (the size of a deck of cards), 1 egg, ½ cup cooked beans, 2 tablespoons peanut butter, ⅓ cup nuts
Milk, yogurt and cheese	2 to 3 servings per day	1 cup low-fat milk or yogurt, 2 ounces cheese, ¾ cup cottage cheese
Grains	5 to 6 servings per day	1 slice whole-grain bread, ½ bagel, ½ cup cooked pasta, rice or hot cereal, 1 ounce ready-to-eat cereal
Fats, oils and sweets	Use sparingly	N/A

Based on the United States Department of Agriculture/U.S. Department of Health and Human Service's Food Guide Pyramid. Amounts assume an 1,800 calorie-per-day diet.

as well as protein and a little fat, while a skinless chicken breast delivers protein and some fat. Depending on how much you know about nutrition, it may be difficult to achieve a perfect balance of protein, fat and carbs at every meal. But you should come close if you follow the basic guidelines of the Food Pyramid.

The Turn Back the Clock Meal Plan on pages 179 to 203 also adheres to these general nutritional principles. Each of the seven daily menus is made up of three smallish meals and two snacks that all contain a healthy balance of carbs, protein and fat. When you see the menus, some of you may think, "Gee, this is more food than I used to eat!" That's the beauty of sensible eating programs like mine. You eat often and fill up with lots of good-for-you foods—there's no such thing as starving.

If you're following the complete Fit and Fabulous Pyramid Plan, you're also burning calories and boosting your metabolism through EXERCISE, so you can afford to eat a little more. Remember: Exercise is an absolute necessity for a healthy heart and lungs as well as a strong, active, pain-free body. And as you know, the basic principle of weight loss is that calories burned must exceed calories consumed. So you must keep moving in order to preserve your body and keep extra pounds at bay.

9 SIMPLE ANTI-AGING STRATEGIES

As we get older, our bodies change. Our metabolism slows down and we gain weight. We start losing bone and muscle at an accelerated rate. We experience symptoms of menopause such as hot flashes. And our immune system starts to weaken, leaving us more vulnerable to colds, influenza and other health-related problems.

While you can't expect to live forever, you *can* use food to fight these natural progressions and turn back the clock. It may sound complicated, but you don't need a Ph.D. in nutrition to minimize middle-age spread and ward off problems like heart disease, osteoporosis, diabetes and cancer. Just follow these nine simple strategies:

1. Keep Tabs on Your Metabolism

Metabolism is the rate at which your body burns calories. Some people are blessed with high metabolic rates (you know who they are—they eat all day and still wear a size 4). The rest of us need to take matters into our own hands, especially as we age.

Your metabolism naturally starts to slow down as you become less active and your body loses muscle. As you found out in Chapter 3, regular aerobic exercise and strength training can help give your metabolism a boost. But how and when you eat also plays an important role. Here are six easy ways to keep your metabolism charged.

Don't skip meals—especially breakfast. Whether you're trying to drop weight quickly or are simply in too much of a hurry, skipping meals is a big mistake. When your body is deprived of food, it starts conserving fuel—in other words, burning fewer calories to protect itself from starving. This is especially bad news for those who don't eat breakfast. Since your body slows down while it's sleeping, you need food to give your metabolism a kick—not to mention to provide energy and brainpower. While a balanced breakfast is best, in a pinch even a modest glass of orange juice and a banana is better than nothing. Breakfast is also a prime opportunity to squeeze in some of those fruit and veggie servings that we'll be talking about later. If you feel hungrier and end up eating more than you used to when you skipped breakfast, that's okay—you're eating more because you're burning more calories. You can afford a little extra!

Healthy Breakfasts on the Run

Breakfast is the most important meal of the day, so you don't want to skip it, even if you're in a rush. What to do? Stock up on healthy breakfast foods that can be eaten in the car, on a bus or train, or at your desk at work while you're checking E-mail. Here, examples of five perfect A.M. pick-me-ups that travel well.

- A cup of low-fat yogurt, a small plastic bag filled with whole-grain cereal and a small container of orange or grapefruit juice
- A soy butter and banana sandwich on whole-grain bread
- Two apple halves topped with reduced-fat natural peanut butter
- A power smoothie made with ice, soy milk or fruit juice, low-fat yogurt, banana and mixed berries
- A whole-grain bagel spread with a thin layer of low-fat cream cheese and sliced cucumbers or tomatoes

Spread your food intake throughout the day. While skipping meals is a definite weight-loss don't, eating too much food at once can also sabotage your efforts to beat middle-age spread. As I mentioned before, your body processes fuel more efficiently when it's fed in small amounts. Several studies show that people who eat consistently and evenly throughout the day tend to have lower levels of body fat than those who sit down to heavy meals. "Grazing" may be the secret to keeping your metabolism revved, your blood sugar stable and your body primed for movement.

I'm not suggesting that you spend a lot more time in the kitchen—just that you make a few timing changes. Instead of eating a sandwich, a piece of fruit and a few Fig Newtons all in one sitting, space them out—a sandwich at noon, an apple at 1:30 and cookies at 3. Rather than eating a three-course dinner, chomp your salad at 5:30 or 6, while your chicken and wild rice are cooking.

The aim is to keep your body fueled for activity and prevent what I call the I'm-starving-so-I'll-stuff-myself-silly problem. We've all been there. We're so hungry that not only will we eat the first thing we see, we eat way too much of it—and, needless to say, regret it later. Eat a banana at 11 A.M., *before* your tummy starts to grumble. Listen to your body's signals and find what works for you.

Since a balanced meal isn't always possible, get in the habit of keeping a nutritious snack in your desk or tote bag. An energy bar shouldn't serve as a meal, but it will keep your engine running until you can sit down to a healthy lunch or dinner.

Watch your portion sizes. America is the land of extra-large everything—from jumbo sodas to super-size fries to overstuffed sandwiches. While we should be eating meals the size of airplane entrées, we're sitting down to salads made with one and a half heads of romaine lettuce or pasta dishes big enough to feed a family of four. According to a recent survey by the American Institute for Cancer Research, most Americans ignore the importance of portion sizes. No wonder we're gaining weight!

The first step in defending yourself against the overeating epidemic? Learn what appropriate serving sizes look like. (See the examples on page 128.) Other tips: If you're eating out at a restaurant, ask your server to put half of your salad or sandwich in a doggie bag when you place your order—before it arrives in front of you. Less temptation! Order soup, then wait and see if you're still hungry. Or split a meal with a friend. Eating large amounts at one sitting overloads your system, which fouls up your digestion *and* adds up to unwanted body fat. Research proves it—so don't do it!

Put a curfew on your kitchen. Does late-night eating make you gain weight? Technically, no. According to top weight loss experts, your body doesn't metabolize food more slowly at night than it does during the day—so a slice of pizza eaten at 9 P.M. is no more likely to land on your hips than one eaten at 6 P.M.

Weight gain happens when you consume more calories than you burn. Period. Unfortunately, late-night nibbling often does set you up for overeating. Mindless munching in front of the TV can add up to a lot of excess calories. Then there are the people who "save up" their calories all day and stuff themselves at night; these folks often eat more in one meal than other people do throughout an entire day.

Besides eating lots of mini-meals to keep my blood sugar stable and prevent pig-outs, I try to eat an early dinner—between 6 and 7 P.M. At 8 P.M. sharp I shut my kitchen doors—after that, it's only water for me. I brush my teeth right away, so I'm not even tempted to dig into the cookies, then take our dog, Madonna, for a walk or watch TV with Jeff. My eight o'clock "curfew" allows me time to digest before going to bed. I sleep better and wake up with a healthy appetite—and that's when I jump-start my metabolism with a nutritious breakfast.

What if you're really hungry late at night? Then eat! Remember, the goal isn't to starve your body, and you don't want to go to bed hungry. Lean protein (white-meat chicken or turkey, low-fat cheese, skim milk) and fibrous fruits and vegetables (apples, oranges, raisins, sweet potatoes, broccoli, green peas) are your best before-bedtime choices. Why? Because they fill you up quickly with relatively few calories, and you're less likely to overeat them than starches like bread and pasta.

2. Combat Free Radicals

Free radicals—we hear lots of talk about these harmful substances. But what are they exactly? Free radicals, found in air pollution, cigarette smoke, fried foods and other unhealthy things, are molecules with unpaired electrons. The free radicals go out in search of that extra electron, and during the search, they attack healthy cells, hoping to "steal" one of theirs. When they do, they leave the healthy cell damaged and defenseless . . . the first step toward many serious diseases, including cancer.

Even if you quit smoking, give up french fries and move to a clean-air state like Alaska, you can't totally avoid free radicals. But you *can* combat them by eating foods rich in antioxidants—namely, fruits and vegetables. Antioxidants can stop free radicals from attacking healthy cells and help keep your body resistant to heart disease, cancer and other undiscriminating killers. Fruits and veggies are also low in calories, so eating them can help you control your weight. Best of all, they're delicious! To me, there is nothing more satisfying than a sweet piece of pineapple or a savory acorn squash.

To keep free radicals at bay, aim to eat at least five and preferably eight servings of fruits and vegetables per day. I can almost hear some of you groaning out there. Don't worry. Getting five to eight servings of fruits and vegetables is easier than it may sound. The reason: Serving sizes are smaller than most people think. A glass of grapefruit juice, a banana and a big handful of blueberries on your breakfast cereal, and you're a third of the way to your goal. Throw in a few tomato slices on your sandwich, a side salad and an apple as a snack, and you're almost done!

See how easy it is? Here are a few more ways to sneak antioxidant-packed fruits and veggies into your diet:

- Stack spinach leaves, red peppers, cucumbers or sprouts on sandwiches.
- When you're boiling pasta, toss in some raw broccoli during the last few minutes, then drain and serve with your favorite sauce.
- Chop an apple and add to instant oatmeal before microwaving. A fresh twist to an old favorite!
- Order a side of steamed or sautéed veggies instead of fries with your sandwich or burger.
- Add lightly steamed fresh or frozen chopped veggies to canned soup.
- Mix orange juice with seltzer or diet lemon-lime soda—my favorite fizzy beverage.
- Top a frozen pizza or entrée with chopped broccoli, carrots, zucchini and other veggies. (Depending on cooking time, you may want to lightly steam certain veggies first.)
- Try a veggie egg-white omelet as an alternative to scrambled or poached eggs.
- Lightly steam fresh or frozen veggies and add to your favorite pasta sauce.
- Snack on celery sticks spread with light tofu "cream cheese."

Eating more fruits and veggies is one of the biggest favors that you can do for your body. Last year, one of my friends—a certified pizza and burgers junkie—made it her New Year's resolution to eat "five a day." She not only dropped weight, she had more energy and swore that her skin looked better than ever. If you have trouble making it work, try mapping out your five to eight servings every morning. Place your veggie servings, washed and ready to eat, in a Tupperware container, then pick out a few pieces of fruit and keep them in a visible place—on the kitchen counter or your desk at work. It's impossible to forget when they're sitting right in front of you!

Fresh? Canned? Frozen? Now You Can Use All Three!

I used to pride myself on using only fresh fruits and vegetables. But now I find that there are frozen and canned foods with just as many nutrients and almost as much flavor as fresh. Fresh produce can take two weeks to get to your supermarket, and it continues to lose nutrients with each day that passes. Most frozen and canned fruits and veggies, on the other hand, are packaged immediately upon harvesting, while they're at their prime. In fact, a recent study conducted by the University of Illinois Department of Food Science and Human Nutrition shows that, in some cases, canned or frozen fruits and vegetables can be *more* nutritious than fresh. I still prefer to eat fresh produce whenever possible—I like the taste and texture better. But in a pinch, frozen or canned fruits and veggies are great, time-saving alternatives—already washed, trimmed and measured for servings. Beware of ones that contain added salt or sugary syrup, but it's easy to find frozen produce that doesn't have these additives. If you're using canned goods, opt for low-sodium vegetables and fruits packed in juice or light syrup and drain well before eating.

3. Take Supplements

When it comes to vitamin and mineral supplements, I tend to be a minimalist. If you eat a healthy diet filled with fruits and vegetables (which I generally do), top researchers have told me, you can get all the nutrients you need from food. But no matter how well you eat, they say, it's wise to pop a multivitamin as an insurance policy.

A good multivitamin will provide at least 100 percent of the recommended daily allowance (RDA) for most nutrients, including vitamin A (20 percent or more as beta-carotene), vitamin D, vitamin K and trace minerals (chromium, copper, manganese, selenium, zinc). With a few possible exceptions (which I'll talk about in a minute), your body doesn't need more than the RDA. In fact, taking too much of certain fat-soluble nutrients such as vitamins A, D and K could cause problems ranging from skin rash to liver damage.

In addition to a multivitamin, I also take a daily calcium supplement. Most multiples fall way short of the RDA for this bone-building mineral (they'd be the size of a golf ball if they didn't), so experts recommend taking a separate supplement to make sure that your calcium needs are met. Aim for one that contains at least 500 mg of calcium. (I'll explain more about this important mineral on page 135.)

If your multiple doesn't supply 250 to 1,000 mg of vitamin C and 100 to 400 IU of vitamin E, you may want to consider taking more of those nutrients as well. Vitamin C is a powerful antioxidant that has been linked to enhanced immune function and lower risk of cataracts. Some studies also suggest that vitamin E can help lower your risk of heart disease by preventing the buildup of fatty plaque on artery walls. While taking extra doses of these antioxidant vitamins should help rather than hurt you, be sure to ask your physician about it to get his or her take.

If you're ever wondering whether to take more of certain vitamins or thinking about experimenting with herbs such as St. John's wort or ginseng, always talk to your doctor first. Because of the danger of unpleasant side effects and harmful drug interactions, it's important to get an expert opinion before popping anything—especially herbal supplements. Vitamins and herbs aren't regulated by any government agency, and there haven't been a lot of studies to monitor the long-term benefits and side effects—so it's anyone's guess whether that pill you're taking is truly effective or will cause other problems further down the road.

One other tip: Keep your vitamin and mineral supplements visible, not hidden. I keep my bottles in a kitchen cupboard with the drinking glasses. Every morning when I open up the cupboard to get a glass, I'm reminded to pop those pills. The more you see them, the more likely you are to take them!

You'll learn more about different nutrients and their benefits on the following pages. Meanwhile, don't forget that taking a supplement isn't an excuse to skip nutritional foods!

Denise's Daily Dose

Basic multivitamin
500–1,000 mg of calcium
500 mg of vitamin C
400 IU of vitamin E

4. Bone Up on Calcium

Drink your milk. You heard it constantly as a kid, and for good reason. The calcium found in milk is essential for building and maintaining strong bones. Without it, your bones can become thin, brittle and at risk for fractures—a condition called osteoporosis, which afflicts half of all American women over age 65.

Most women reach their peak bone density in their late 20s. After that, depending on our genetics and our lifestyle, many of us start losing bone at a very slow rate. The female hormone estrogen helps us maintain our bone density, so when we hit menopause and estrogen production stops, the rate of bone loss often escalates. According to the National Osteoporosis Foundation, some women lose up to 20 percent of their bone mass in the five to seven years following menopause.

Women have smaller, more fragile skeletons to begin with, putting us at greater risk for osteoporosis than men (though men suffer from it, too). Factor in years of poor eating habits, lack of exercise, smoking or too much boozing, and our bones really pay the price.

Supplemental Knowledge

In an ideal world, we would receive all of our vitamins and minerals from the food we eat. Unfortunately, few of us have the knowledge, patience and time to create perfect meals every day, so supplements are an important nutritional aid. Use the charts below to learn more about what you should be taking and why.

Vitamins

Unlike protein, carbohydrates and fat, vitamins aren't sources of energy. But these organic micronutrients are essential for energy metabolism, cell production, bone formation and overall good health. There are two types of vitamins: fat soluble and water soluble. Water-soluble vitamins (vitamin C and the B vitamins, including biotin, folate and panothenic acid) are utilized by your body very quickly; excess amounts are excreted in your urine. Fat-soluble vitamins (vitamins A, D, E and K) are used up very slowly and can be stored in your liver and body fat; they have the potential to be toxic, so watch your intake. Unless otherwise noted, optimal intakes are based on the Recommended Daily Allowances for women set by the National Academy of Sciences–National Research Council.

Vitamin	Optimal Intake	What It Can Do	Where You Can Find It
A	4,000 IU	Promote good eyesight as well as healthy skin, bones and teeth; protect against heart disease; boost immunity; help minimize wrinkles and age spots	Carrots; dark green and yellow vegetables; orange fruits; eggs; milk; cheese
B_1 (THIAMINE)	1.1 mg	Keep nervous system, heart and muscles functioning normally; improve mood and mental attitude; combat motion sickness	Whole grains; oatmeal; peanuts; lean pork; most vegetables; milk; seeds
B_2 (RIBOFLAVIN)	1.1 mg	Promote healthy skin, nails and hair; improve vision and relieve eye fatigue	Milk, yogurt; dark, leafy greens; eggs; cheese; whole grains

Vitamin	Optimal Intake	What It Can Do	Where You Can Find It
B$_3$ (NIACIN)	Under age 50: 1.3 mg Over age 50: 1.5 mg	Promote healthy skin; aid digestion; lower high blood pressure; boost energy; relieve canker sores	Lean pork; swordfish; mackerel; chicken; whole-grain breads and cereals; wheat germ; fish; eggs; milk; nuts; peanut butter; avocados; dates; figs; prunes
B$_6$	14 mg	Promote new cell growth; help regulate blood sugar; boost immunity; improve nerve function and memory; may help lower risk of heart attack or stroke	Wheat germ; soybeans; cantaloupe; mangos; lean meat and poultry; eggs; oats; peanuts; walnuts; lentils; green leafy vegetables
B$_{12}$	2.4 mcg	Increase production of red blood cells; promote a healthy nervous system; boost energy; improve concentration, memory and balance	Meat; fish; eggs; milk; cheese; clams
BIOTIN	30 mcg	Ease muscle pains; alleviate skin conditions such as eczema and dermatitis; may keep hair from turning gray	Egg yolks; soy flour; brewer's yeast; milk

Vitamin	Optimal Intake	What It Can Do	Where You Can Find It
C	75 mg	Aid in collagen production, which is necessary for healthy blood vessels, bones, teeth, gums and skin; help lower blood cholesterol; boost immune system	Citrus fruits; kiwis; berries; green leafy vegetables; melon; mangos; broccoli; tomatoes; red peppers; potatoes
CHOLINE	425 mg	Aid in the transmittal of nerve impulses to enhance memory; maintain liver health; help prevent heart disease by clearing excessive levels of homocysteine from your blood	Milk; eggs; beef; peanuts; whole-grain bread; cauliflower; oranges
D	Under age 50: 200 IU Ages 51 to 70: 400 IU Over age 70: 600 IU	Increase calcium absorption and utilization, which translates to strong bones and teeth	Tuna; salmon; sardines; herring; fortified milk and dairy products (also derived from exposing skin to the sun)
E	30 IU	Lower risk of cardiovascular disease; enhance immunity; aid in formation of red blood cells, muscles and tissues; minimize signs of sun damage	Vegetable oils; sweet potatoes; avocados; dark leafy greens; Brussels sprouts; nuts; peanut butter; wheat germ; whole-grain cereals; eggs

Vitamin	Optimal Intake	What It Can Do	Where You Can Find It
FOLATE (FOLIC ACID)	400 mcg	Promote healthy skin; improve concentration and mood; aid in digestion; prevent some birth defects; protect against heart attack and stroke	Fortified cereals; beans; dark leafy greens; carrots; avocados; asparagus; oranges; cantaloupe; apricots; pumpkin
K	65 mcg	Promote proper blood clotting; help maintain healthy bones and heal fractures	Canola, safflower and soybean oils; broccoli; kale; spinach; cabbage; cauliflower; bran; egg yolks
PANTOTHENIC ACID	5 mg	Essential for normal cell development and growth; helps convert sugar and fat into energy; aids in wound healing; prevents fatigue	Meat; whole grains; wheat germ; bran; green vegetables; nuts; chicken

Minerals

Like vitamins, minerals are also micronutrients. The difference is that most minerals are inorganic, meaning they don't come from either animals or vegetables. Minerals play a key role in the activation of hormones and enzymes and the formation of tissues and bones. There are more than 22 known minerals, but I've outlined the most important ones here.

Mineral	Optimal Intake	What It Can Do	Where You Can Find It
CALCIUM	1,000–1,500 mg	Help build and maintain healthy bones and teeth	Milk, yogurt; cheese; tofu; salmon; dark, leafy greens; beans; figs; fortified cereal and orange juice

Mineral	Optimal Intake	What It Can Do	Where You Can Find It
CHROMIUM	120 mcg	Help maintain normal blood sugar levels; prevent and lower high blood pressure; may help build strong muscles and minimize fat storage	Whole-grain breads and cereals; wheat germ; brewer's yeast; chicken; cheese
COPPER	2 mg	Aid in iron absorption; increase energy	Beans; peas; whole-grain cereals and breads; prunes; seafood
IODINE	150 mcg	Help regulate the thyroid gland, which can boost energy and control weight; promote healthy hair, skin, nails and teeth	Kelp; onions; seafood
IRON	15 mg premenopause; 10 mg postmenopause	Deliver oxygen to muscles to help prevent fatigue; increase resistance to disease; promote healthy skin tone and color	Lean meats such as pork and poultry; eggs; oysters; beans; lentils; nuts; dark leafy greens; oatmeal
MAGNESIUM	320 mg	Promote a healthy heart and cardiovascular system; combat depression; maintain healthy teeth; prevent kidney stones and gallstones; relieve indigestion	Dark leafy greens; nuts; soybeans; seafood; wheat germ; whole-grain cereals and breads

Mineral	Optimal Intake	What It Can Do	Where You Can Find It
MANGANESE	2 mg	Help reduce fatigue; improve memory; aid in muscle reflexes; reduce nervous irritability	Whole-grain cereals; nuts; dark leafy greens; peas; beets
POTASSIUM	2,000 mg	Aid in proper muscle function; minimize soreness after exercise; increase concentration and clarity by sending oxygen to the brain; help reduce high blood pressure	Bananas; citrus fruits; cantaloupe; apricots; tomatoes; sunflower seeds; potatoes; mint leaves
PHOSPHORUS	1,000 mg	Aid in growth and repair of cells; increase energy; promote healthy gums and teeth; minimize arthritis pain	Fish; poultry; meat; whole grains; eggs; nuts; seeds
SELENIUM	70 mcg	Slow down aging and hardening of tissues; alleviate hot flashes; possibly help protect against certain cancers	Seafood; wheat germ; bran; tuna; onions; tomatoes; broccoli
ZINC	12 mg	Enhance immune system; aid in proper muscle contraction; boost mental alertness; improve sexual function; help decrease cholesterol deposits	Oysters; herring; milk; red meat; poultry; eggs

Herbs

Herbal "medicines" are everywhere: in pill form and in your favorite iced tea, snack food and soup. What are these natural "wonder drugs" and do they work? The simple answer is that we don't know yet. Some people swear by herbs, but more scientific research is needed to prove that they offer any healing benefit. Meanwhile, herbal products aren't regulated by the Food and Drug Administration or any other government agency, meaning there's no way to tell whether they're safe or effective. The long-term effects simply haven't been studied. If you're interested in trying one of these remedies, discuss it with your doctor first. If you're taking any prescription or over-the-counter medications, there is the potential for dangerous interactions and side effects. At the very least, you should talk to your pharmacist and check the following Web sites for updated information: www.fda.gov (Food and Drug Administration) and www.nnfa.com (National Nutritional Food Association).

Here is a list of some popular herbs available today:

Herb	What It Does	Dos and Don'ts
BLACK COHOSH	Relieves PMS and meno-pause symptoms; reduces high blood pressure	Use with physician approval and supervision only
ECHINACEA	Boosts immunity and fights the common cold	Use in consultation with a doctor; stop using or lower dose if you experi-ence stomach upset or diarrhea
EPHEDRA	Acts as a natural stimu-lant; opens bronchial passages; increases blood pressure, metabolic rate, perspiration and urine production	Use only in consultation with a physician; do not use if you have high blood pressure, heart dis-ease, diabetes, glaucoma or an overactive thyroid
GINGKO BILOBA	Enhances memory and reaction time; improves blood flow to the heart; reduces the risk of blood clots	Use only in consultation with a doctor; avoid if you take aspirin, ticlopidine (Ticlid) or dipyridamole (Persantine)

Herb	What It Does	Dos and Don'ts
GINSENG	Boosts mental and physical energy; relieves indigestion and insomnia; improves circulation	Generally considered safe; don't use if you have a fever, asthma, high blood pressure or cardiac arrhythmia; use with caution if you have insomnia, hay fever or fibrocystic breasts
KAVA KAVA	Relieves stress, tension, anxiety and sleeplessness	Use in consultation with your doctor; don't use if you're taking sleeping pills, antipsychotic medication, drugs for Parkinson's or when you drink alcohol
ST. JOHN'S WORT	Fights depression and SAD (seasonal affective disorder)	Use in consultation with your doctor; don't take if you're already on a type of antidepressant known as MAO inhibitors or if you're taking diet pills, asthma inhalants, nasal decongestants, or cold or hay fever medications; it can reduce the effectiveness of birth control pills, so check with your doctor

Calcium consumption is very important during childhood and into your 20s, when bones continue to strengthen and grow. But even after that, a calcium-rich diet can help prevent the bone loss that leads to debilitating fractures. Studies have shown that women who consume more than 760 mg of calcium daily reduce their risk of hip fractures by up to 60 percent.

Experts recommend consuming about 1,000 mg of calcium per day before menopause; 1,200 to 1,500 mg during pregnancy and breastfeeding; 1,500 mg for postmenopausal women who *aren't* on hormone replacement therapy; and 1,000 mg for women who *are* on hormone replacement therapy.

Milk and dairy products are rich sources of this bone-building mineral. But there are many other options for women who are lactose intolerant or who simply don't like dairy foods. Tofu, soybeans and leafy green vegetables such as spinach and kale are excellent choices. Figs and beans are also rich in calcium.

Calcium isn't the only weapon against osteoporosis. Vitamin D and magnesium are integral, since they help your body absorb bone-fortifying calcium. Milk is an excellent source of vitamin D, and so are fishes like salmon, tuna and sardines. The sun can also be a good source of vitamin D, but you need to be extremely careful to protect yourself from damaging ultraviolet rays that can cause skin cancer and premature aging. (Always wear sunblock with an SPF of 15 or higher. Otherwise 15 to 20 minutes without sunblock and about 30 percent of your body not covered with clothes gets a healthy dose of vitamin D.) Magnesium can be found in foods such as dark leafy greens, soybeans, wheat germ and fortified cereal.

No matter how healthy your diet, supplements are also strongly advised. Most multivitamins contain only a fraction of the recommended daily dose of calcium, so it's a good idea to take a separate calcium supplement (that's what I do). There's a wide range of calcium supplements to choose from, including pills, Tums and chocolate chews from Viactiv (my personal favorite—honestly, they taste like candy).

Aside from eating a diet rich in bone-building nutrients, there are other important steps that you should take to protect your bones—namely, stop smoking and cut back on your alcohol intake. Exercise is also essential in the fight against osteoporosis: In a recent six-year study conducted at Pennsylvania State University College of Medicine, researchers found that girls who exercised regularly (nearly every day) had the strongest bones. New research from the University of Arkansas

10 Super Sources of Calcium

Yogurt, plain, nonfat (1 cup)	400–450 mg
Yogurt, flavored, nonfat (1 cup)	314–350 mg
Skim milk (1 cup)	300 mg
Tofu (4 ounces or ½ cup)	258 mg
Calcium-fortified orange juice (¾ cup)	225 mg
Cheddar cheese (1 ounce)	204 mg
Total cereal (1 ounce)	200 mg
Ricotta cheese, part skim (¼ cup)	169 mg
Collard greens (½ cup)	150 mg
Broccoli (½ cup)	89 mg
Spinach (½ cup)	84 mg
White beans (½ cup)	80 mg
Cottage cheese (4 ounces)	77 mg

Easy Ways to Boost Your Calcium

- Buy calcium-fortified orange juice.

- Add nonfat dry milk powder to baked goods, mashed potatoes or meat-balls.

- Make a shake using nonfat milk, soy milk (fortified with calcium and vita-min D), fresh fruit and yogurt.

- For a healthy dessert, top vanilla yogurt with fresh berries.

- Add milk instead of water to your morning instant oatmeal.

- Skip a green salad and go for sautéed spinach or broccoli—both contain calcium.

- Toss white beans into your favorite pasta.

- Try frozen tofu lasagna—several food manufacturers, including Amy's Kitchen, make it!

- Place a broiled chicken breast on a bed of collard greens or spinach instead of pasta.

- Warm up with a nonfat chai tea latte (a blend of different teas).

also suggests that gardening helps increase bone density in women over age 50. So get out there and walk, jog, play golf, rake the lawn or water your flowers—your bones will thank you!

5. Fill Up with Fiber

You've known that fiber is good for your body ever since you saw your great-aunt Alberta drinking murky prune juice. But it may be even better for you than you think. Besides keeping you "regular," a diet rich in fiber may help protect your heart, your waistline and your smile.

New research shows that a diet rich in soluble fiber, found in dried beans and peas, fruits and vegetables, oats and flax, can significantly lower your risk of heart disease, the leading cause of death among women. In a study published in the *Journal of the American Medical Association*, women who consumed the most soluble fiber were 23 percent less likely to suffer heart attacks than those who consumed the least. This is largely because foods rich in soluble fiber help drive down LDL cholesterol levels. (Remember the oat bran craze of the early 90s? It wasn't so crazy—it really works!)

Fiber can also help you lose weight by making you feel full, so you eat less overall—a natural appetite suppressant! According to a U.S.

15 Fabulous Fiber Sources

Raisin bran cereal (¾ cup)	4.5–8.0 grams
Sweet potato, 1 medium	7.2 grams
Raisins (½ cup)	4.3 grams
Spinach, cooked (1 cup)	4 grams
Blackberries (½ cup)	3.7 grams
Apple, 1 medium	3.4 grams
Black beans (½ cup)	2.4 grams
White beans (½ cup)	2.2 grams
Oat bran, cooked (¾ cup)	2.2 grams
Kidney beans (½ cup)	2.0 grams
Brussels sprouts (½ cup)	2.0 grams
Apricots (4)	1.8 grams
Orange (1)	1.8 grams
Mango (½)	1.7 grams
Turnips (½ cup)	1.7 grams

Department of Agriculture study published in the *Journal of Nutrition*, fiber also whisks food through your digestive system before it can be absorbed and stored as fat. (While you also may lose some vitamins and minerals during this process, the researchers say that those losses can be minimized if your fiber comes from a variety of foods—whole grains, fruits and vegetables—instead of a single source such as bran cereal.) Another bonus is that crunchy, fiber-filled foods such as nuts, raw carrots and apples help keep your teeth and gums healthy, so you'll be less likely to develop periodontal disease.

Nutrition experts recommend consuming at least 25 to 30 grams of fiber per day, but the average American woman only gets about half that amount. With all the benefits of fiber, we need to work hard to add it to our daily eating plans!

6. Drink from the Water Fountain of Youth

Water is truly a miracle drink. Your body needs it for countless behind-the-scenes processes, from digesting food to regulating body temperature. Even though it doesn't contain calories, water contributes to a feeling of fullness, making it an excellent weight-loss aid. Feeling fatigued? You may not need sleep—you could simply be dehydrated. Many women walk around in a mild state of dehydration, which means your blood volume is lowered. That results in less blood getting to your brain and your heart has to pump harder. By the time you actually feel thirsty, you've already lost *2 to 3 percent of your body fluid.*

Trade in Fiber-Free for Fiber-Full Foods!

Getting the recommended 25 to 30 grams of fiber a day can be easily accomplished with a few simple dietary switches—no prunes required!

BREAKFAST

Instead of:	1 cup cornflakes (1 gram fiber)
Choose:	½ cup Fiber One cereal (13 grams fiber)
Instead of:	White bread (0–1 gram fiber)
Choose:	Whole-wheat bread (2–3 grams fiber)
Instead of:	6 ounces orange juice (0 grams fiber)
Choose:	1 orange (3 grams fiber)

LUNCH

Instead of:	A cheeseburger (0 grams fiber)
Choose:	Black-bean burger (4.8 grams fiber)
Instead of:	1 cup chicken noodle soup (2 grams fiber)
Choose:	1 cup lentil soup (5 grams fiber)
Instead of:	Turkey sandwich on a hard roll (1 gram fiber)
Choose:	⅓ cup hummus on a whole-wheat pita (9 grams fiber)

SNACKS

Instead of:	Potato chips (0 grams fiber)
Choose:	Baked tortilla chips with salsa (2.2 grams fiber)
Instead of:	Cheese curls (0 grams fiber)
Choose:	Popcorn (4.7 grams fiber)
Instead of:	Gummi Bears (0 grams fiber)
Choose:	Dried apricots (4 grams fiber)

DINNER

Instead of:	Marinara sauce (3 grams fiber)
Choose:	Chunky vegetable sauce (6 grams fiber)
Instead of:	Two-thirds cup white rice (0 grams fiber)
Choose:	Two-thirds cup brown rice (2.3 grams fiber)
Instead of:	Grilled chicken (0 grams fiber)
Choose:	Veggie burger (4 grams fiber)

Are you drinking enough H_2O? One way to tell is to check the color of your urine. If it's a very pale yellow, you're fine; if it's bright yellow or deep gold, you need to drink more. Another simple hydration test: Pinch the skin on the back of your hand. If it springs back into place quickly, you should be sufficiently hydrated. If not, it's time to reach for a water bottle!

Always aim to drink *at least* 8 to 10 glasses of water a day (even more when you exercise or consume alcohol or caffeinated beverages). I like to carry a water bottle around with me everywhere I go; I also keep

The Best Drinks in the House

As I discuss later, coffee, cola and other caffeinated beverages are diuretics, meaning they increase the flow of urine from your body. While they may quench your thirst temporarily, they ultimately rob water from your system, leaving you even more dehydrated than before—not to mention constantly running for the bathroom. Water is always your best beverage choice with meals, but if you do decide to have a cup of coffee or a diet cola, try to accompany it with a glass of H_2O. If you get tired of plain water, here are some variations that might inspire you:

Ice water with lemon, lime or orange slices

Seltzer with a splash of cranberry, grapefruit or lime juice

Flavored seltzer or Perrier

Iced tea (decaffeinated) with a sprig of fresh mint (preferably sweetened)

Green tea

Sugar-free Tang

spares in my car and in my gym bag. Other great get-more-water strategies: Drink a big glass or two as soon as you get up in the morning and before each meal, then sip as you eat. Not only will you find yourself satisfied with smaller portions, you'll be done with your daily quota before you know it.

Need more incentive? Picture a prune. Yes, that shriveled-up piece of fruit is actually a dehydrated plum. When we don't get enough fluids, the same thing happens to our bodies' cells and tissues—hello, wrinkles! Or think of the news stories that we've all seen about men and women who are rescued after days without water. They look like they've aged overnight. Sure, it's the stress—but it's also a lack of proper fluids and nourishment. Our bodies need water. So drink up!

7. Limit Processed and Sugary Foods

Here's a confession: I love junk food. I love donuts and potato chips and ice cream and even the occasional slice of rich, gooey chocolate cake. Katie and Kelly do, too—and sometimes when I'm around them, I just can't resist. Those cravings for sinful sweets, salty snacks and other nutritional zeroes happen to everyone. And there *is* room in our diet for splurges. The key isn't eliminating these treats—it's learning to enjoy them in moderation.

Nutrition experts say that less than 10 percent of your calories should come from sugary, processed foods; for an 1,800-calorie-per-day diet, that's under 180 calories. The reasons are obvious. If you're worried about your weight, those extra calories can add up. (Just think: 10 jelly beans, 2 Hershey's Kisses and a Coke have as many calories as a light frozen entrée plus a fruit dessert—and which do you think is more satisfying?) And if you're filling up on junk, you're probably missing out on important nutrients that will keep you healthy and fit as you grow older.

The other problem with sweets is that they're addictive. Sure, you can't compare cookies and ice cream to nicotine, but some researchers maintain that the taste of refined sugar creates a yearning for more refined sugar. The more you eat, the more you want. And most sugary foods (such as candy, frozen yogurt and cola) are devoid of fiber, so you're left feeling empty and unsatisfied—and you just keep eating.

The next time you pick up a candy bar, check out the nutritional label. Chances are that small bar has well over 200 calories. Why blow all your sugar calories in one fell swoop? Instead, bite into a delicious piece of fresh fruit, nibble some dried apricots or put a few tiny chocolate chips on some nonfat yogurt. Your sweet tooth will be satisfied and so will some of your nutritional needs.

A juicy plum or chewy apricots may not sound as tempting, but as soon as it's in your mouth, you may be surprised at how much you enjoy your healthful snack—and how you don't miss the old "empty" one at all. A nutritious snack will boost your energy, while junk food zaps it. So when you're trying to choose between a crunchy apple and a chocolate chip cookie, try to think about how you'll feel afterward. I find it makes the decision much easier!

Remember: Don't beat yourself up if you succumb to a crème brûlée or just can't resist a chocolate chip cookie (or two!). You're allowed to enjoy yourself and indulge in the delectable treats every now and then—I certainly do. Besides, denying yourself your favorite foods can lead to binges. As long as you're getting your fill of nutrient-dense foods and aren't going overboard on junk, you'll be in good shape. You

Smart Swaps

It's okay to cave in to your sweet tooth once in a while—everyone needs an occasional treat! But if you can't keep your hands out of the candy or cookie jar, you should try to find healthier, less-fattening ways to satisfy your cravings. Here are some of my favorites.

- Craving candy? Try raisins, an apple or a banana.
- Craving ice cream? Try yogurt with fresh fruit, a soy smoothie or frozen grapes.
- Craving a frozen coffee drink? Try an iced latte made with skim milk or a nonfat cappuccino sprinkled with vanilla.
- Craving chocolate? Try a chocolate ice pop or lollipop.
- Craving cookies? Try a peppermint—or brushing your teeth!

Junk Food Offensive

The best defense is always a good offense, so try these simple strategies to reduce your daily intake of nutritional zeroes. They work for me!

Think mini. Beat your urge to overeat by buying snacks like chips, pretzels, cookies and raisins in single-serving packages.

Go for the Godiva. Indulge your sweet tooth with an expensive piece of "designer" chocolate instead of a convenience-store candy bar. As you eat, close your eyes and savor each tiny nibble. Your taste buds will think "treat" and you will think "reward" for all the good healthy things you've done!

Check the label. Many breakfast cereals, granola bars and other healthy-sounding foods actually contain a lot of added sugar. Watch for ingredients such as corn syrup, fructose, sucrose and dextrose. If these items are listed near the top of the ingredient list on the nutritional label, switch to another brand. Most food stores now offer a wide variety of healthy, low-sugar cereals.

Don't leave home without good-for-you food. You know the feeling: You're at the mall or stuck in the car when you get the munchies or a pang of hunger strikes. The solution: Keep an emergency bag of dried fruit, an apple, an energy bar (preferably one that's lower in sugar) or even a little box of healthy cereal in your purse, pocket or glove compartment. If you're at work, pick up an extra small green salad or container of fruit when you go to lunch, so you can have it on hand for that late-afternoon crash.

Get busy. Boredom can be one of your waistline's worst enemies! It's amazing how you forget to reach for the cookies and candy when you're running around being productive. Use listless moments to do all the things that you've been meaning to do. If your hands are busy writing a letter or scrubbing the tub, they'll be less likely to find their way into the chips and cookies. If that oral fixation resurfaces, try sugar-free gum or hard candy, carrot sticks or apple slices.

can always compensate for it by eating extra well the next day (or, if it's holiday time, the following week). Or get out there and burn off the extra calories by going for a brisk walk or spending a little extra time at the gym. That's my own proactive approach!

8. Avoid Coffee, Cola and Caffeinated Tea (and Be Wrinkle-Free)

Americans love their coffee, and the early-morning latte or cappuccino has become a ritual for millions of women who crave the exotic flavor and the energy boost it brings to their day. Unfortunately, the caffeine found in coffee and certain teas and soft drinks robs your body of the water it needs to be exercise-ready and maintain a supple complexion. And while a cup of coffee or caffeinated tea certainly won't cause harm, I recommend limiting your intake of caffeinated beverages as much as possible—no more than two servings per day.

If you can't live without your coffee or diet cola, don't worry—you can consume extra water to compensate for what your body is losing. On top of your daily 8 to 10 glasses of water, you'll want to down at least one extra 8-ounce glass for each caffeinated drink consumed. In other words, if you drink two cups of coffee, you should aim to drink 10 to 12 glasses of water each day. I know it sounds like a lot, but trust me—it's worth it.

Also, if you're lightening your coffee with cream or milk, or drinking lattes and regular colas, you'll need to watch your calories. A tablespoon of heavy cream contains 52 calories and 5.5 grams of total fat (3.5 grams of artery-damaging saturated fat); an 8-ounce latte (made with 4 ounces of whole milk) delivers about 80 calories and 4 fat grams (2.5 grams of saturated fat); a can of cola has approximately 150 calories. Talk about a real eye-opener!

Another big reason that I limit my intake of coffee, tea and cola: These drinks can stain your teeth, making you look older than your years. When I need a cold refreshment other than water, I reach for a light-colored soft drink, such as 7-Up or Fresca, rather than cola.

I still love my morning cup of coffee, but it would probably be best if I quit. (I just can't give it up!) If you've decided to try to kick your caffeine addiction, your best bet is to wean yourself off these drinks slowly. Gradually reduce your intake by about half a cup every few days. If you try to go cold turkey, you could experience withdrawal symptoms, like a headache or moodiness, that are bound to send you racing toward the first Starbucks you see.

9. Decline Too Much Beer and Wine

Maybe you've heard recent news stories saying that alcoholic beverages can have health benefits; other reports warn against the hazards of drinking wine and booze. Which is correct?

The truth is, it depends. Research indicates that for some people, drinking moderate amounts of alcohol, and wine in particular, may help protect against heart disease, the number-one killer of both men and women. But the key word is *moderation*. For women, "moderate" is defined as no more than *one drink* (a 5-ounce glass of wine, a 12-ounce beer or 1.5 ounces of hard liquor) per day; for men, it's no more than two drinks daily.

Cheers Checklist

If you decide to imbibe, here are some tips before raising your glass:

- If you're drinking at home, buy a small bottle of wine; avoid opening a big bottle, especially if you're the only one indulging!

- Try nonalcoholic wine or beer; it's usually lower in calories, and you won't experience the buzz that can make your appetite spiral out of control. This is a great choice if your doctor advises you to limit your alcohol consumption.

- To combat dehydration, sip water or seltzer along with your alcoholic beverage, and be sure to have at least one big glass of H_2O before or after each cocktail.

But don't assume that if one glass of wine is good for you, two will be better. While one alcoholic drink may help your heart, some studies show that it could increase your risk of breast cancer ever so slightly. Since you're much more likely to get heart disease than breast cancer, many experts say that the gamble might be worth it as long as you stick to one drink. But drinking more alcohol than that is a bad idea, since any potential heart benefits will be overshadowed by a higher risk of breast cancer and liver damage. (And let's face it—we just don't bounce back from a hangover the way we did in our 20s.)

For other people—specifically, anyone with a drinking problem or a family history of alcohol abuse, women who are pregnant or trying to conceive and people taking certain medications—even a small amount of alcohol is ill-advised. My advice: If you fall into any of these categories or if you're at all concerned, talk to your doctor.

Bear in mind that alcohol contains a significant amount of calories. If you're trying to ward off middle-age spread, I suggest keeping tabs on your intake of alcoholic drinks. You don't need to go cold turkey, but remember that the calories can add up quickly. At the very least, alcohol softens our resolve to make healthy food choices.

Finally, like caffeine, alcohol acts as a diuretic, flushing water and vital nutrients out of your system; if your body gets dehydrated, you may feel too tired to work out and your skin will appear dull and wrinkled. Alcohol may also interfere with your sleep patterns. Personally, I like to save my glass of wine for special occasions rather than indulging every evening. But ultimately the decision is yours to make.

The 9 Anti-Aging Strategies Cheat Sheet

1. **Keep tabs on your metabolism**

   - Don't skip meals, especially breakfast

   - Spread your food intake throughout the day

   - Watch your portion sizes

   - Put a curfew on your kitchen

2. **Combat free radicals**

   - Eat 5 to 8 servings of fruits and veggies per day

3. **Take supplements**

   - A basic multivitamin, plus extra calcium and possibly more of vitamins C and E

4. **Bone up on calcium**

   - Get 1,000 mg per day if you're premenopausal or on hormone replacement therapy (HRT)

   - Get 1,500 mg per day if you're postmenopausal and not on HRT

5. **Fill up with fiber**

   - Aim for 25 to 30 grams daily

6. **Drink from the water fountain of youth**

   - Consume at least 8 to 10 glasses of water per day

7. **Limit processed and sugary foods**

   - Less than 10 percent of your calories should come from sugar (fewer than 180 calories for an 1,800-calorie-per-day diet)

8. **Avoid coffee, cola and caffeinated tea (and be wrinkle-free)**

9. **Decline too much beer and wine**

   - Don't exceed one alcoholic beverage a day

THE 10 ULTIMATE AGE-DEFYING FOODS

The best way to achieve optimal nutrition is to eat a wide variety of foods. While it's easy to go with what you know and fill up your grocery cart with old favorites, you can tantalize your taste buds and transform the nutrient profile of your diet by experimenting with new foods. On the following pages I've listed 10 nutritional powerhouses that have been shown through research to have special anti-aging benefits, ranging from protection against heart disease to better vision. I've made an effort to incorporate them into my diet—and you'll want to as well.

1. Soy

If you haven't already, now is the time to stop resisting soy. Research shows that this wonder food can help reduce levels of "bad" LDL cholesterol. Soybeans also contain phytoestrogens called isoflavones that have estrogen-like effects on the body. For menopausal women, this may help minimize hot flashes. The calcium in soybeans also may help reduce your risk of osteoporosis.

More research is needed to know how much soy is needed to alleviate the symptoms of menopause, but studies show that 25 grams of soy protein per day is what it takes to lower cholesterol. That's the equivalent of ½ cup of soy milk (3.5 grams of soy protein), 1 ounce of soy nuts (10.5 grams), 1 ounce of soy cheese (6 grams) and 2 tablespoons of soy nut butter (6 grams). But even if you consume less, you can cut your intake of saturated fat and cholesterol by including more soy and other plant-based sources of protein in your diet.

Perhaps the only women who won't want to pile their plates with soy are those with a personal or family history of estrogen-receptive-positive breast tumors. Since soy seems to mimic estrogen in your body, experts aren't sure what effect it will have on breast tumors. Until more research is done, high-risk women should limit their intake of soy, advises Kim Galeaz, R.D., a nutrition consultant for the United Soybean Board.

Even if you're sold on the benefits of tofu and other soy products, many of you may still be wary—will you ever learn to actually like it? And will you ever get your family to eat it? The answer is yes—I managed to do it, and I've got a houseful of picky eaters! I started by crumbling textured soy protein (which can be found in most supermarkets) into pasta sauces and throwing tiny pieces of tofu into stir-fries. I told the girls that they were eating turkey and chicken, and they gobbled it up. Now we've graduated to soy hot dogs. The kids think that they're eating regular hot dogs, only a different color. Not the most honest approach, but I doubt that they would have eaten them otherwise.

Truth be told, tofu is practically flavorless—it merely soaks up the flavor of whatever sauce or oil it's cooked in. For my family, the spongy texture is what's tough to swallow. But you can disguise it by cutting it up into tiny pieces and adding it to thick stews or sauces Or, start with more palatable soy products such as these:

Edamame: These boiled, salted soybeans found in Japanese restaurants are delicious sources of protein. Nowadays they can be purchased fresh or frozen in many supermarkets as well as specialty food stores. To prepare, you simply steam or boil the soybeans in their pods for no more than 5 minutes. Then lightly salt them and they're ready to eat. Open the pod and pick out the soybeans, or place the whole pod in your mouth and suck out the beans. You'll be amazed—they are every bit as yummy as chips or popcorn! My girls love them.

Miso: A thick paste made from soybeans, sea salt and water, miso is sold in Asian markets as well as most supermarkets. It can be used to make miso soup (a staple in most Japanese restaurants), a sauce for grilled fish like tuna, or salad dressing. Try these quick recipes for great salad toppers: Combine 2 tablespoons of miso with vinegar, orange juice, soy sauce, sesame oil and fresh herbs. Combine ⅛ cup miso with ¼ cup rice wine, ¼ cup dijon mustard, ¼ cup of honey, ½ teaspoon low-sodium soy sauce, ⅛ cup of water and ½ teaspoon ground black pepper.

Soy cheese: This faux cheese is made from tofu and comes in flavors like mozzarella and Swiss; a 1-ounce serving has 60 calories, 4 grams of total fat (and only .5 grams of saturated fat) and 6 grams of protein. Try melting it over tomato slices on whole-wheat bread or sprinkling it on pizzas.

Soy flour: Soybeans are roasted and ground into a fine powder with a flour-like consistency. There are three types of soy flour: defatted (natural oils are removed during processing, which allows for a longer shelf life; this is the best one in my book!), lecithinated (soy lecithin is added to the flour to improve its "mixability") and natural (this flour contains all the natural oil and fat found in soybeans, so it can become rancid very quickly). Soy flour is a great addition to any baked product to provide a little extra protein. But don't use too much—soy flour has no gluten and could ruin your Betty Crocker creation. Check the label for specific instructions.

Soy milk: Ground soybeans are mixed with water to form this milky liquid. An average serving of soy milk (about 1 cup) has about 7 grams of protein and no cholesterol, making it an excellent milk alternative.

While traditional soy milk has about 4 grams of fat per serving, many manufacturers make nonfat versions as well as yummy flavors such as chocolate and vanilla.

Soy nuts: Beware—these crunchy, salty nuggets can be hard to put down. And while they're great sources of soy protein (10.5 grams per ounce), you don't want to eat too many. That same ounce of roasted soybeans delivers about 130 calories and 7 grams of total fat (only 1 of which is saturated).

Soy nut butter: It looks almost exactly like creamy peanut butter, but the taste is a little different. Once you get over the fact that it isn't Skippy, you could get hooked on this sweet, nutty, protein-rich spread. Two tablespoons deliver 170 calories, 11 grams of total fat (1.5 grams of saturated fat) and 6 grams of protein. I like it on whole-grain toast for breakfast.

Tempeh: Hailing from Indonesia, tempeh is a meat-like cultured soybean product. It can be prepared the same way as tofu (see next page).

Textured soy protein: This product, which comes in the form of granules, is made from defatted soy flour. The granules have a very chewy texture and must be boiled in water and drained before using. It makes a great addition to pasta sauces and soups.

Sneaky Ways to Get More Soy

- Sprinkle soy nuts on salads or in soups; nibble them as a protein-rich snack.

- Pour soy milk over breakfast cereal or into a fruit smoothie or coffee.

- Spread soy butter on whole-wheat toast.

- Bake soy flour into muffins.

- Crumble textured soy protein into pasta sauce, chili and stews.

- Toss tofu cubes into stir-fries and soups; scramble into eggs; marinate in soy sauce and ginger, then grill until golden brown; mix with low-fat ricotta cheese for use in stuffed shells or lasagna.

- Trade your chicken cutlet for a vegetarian burger made with soy.

- Order a vegetarian dish with tofu instead of chicken lo mein.

Tofu: Made from boiled, crushed soybeans, tofu comes in thick blocks that can be sliced or chopped. It's a delicious addition to a vegetable stir-fry or pasta sauce, or marinated in soy sauce and ginger and then grilled. I also make tofu enchiladas and faijitas. Try it in any dish that normally calls for chicken.

2. Fish

Fish, especially fatty fish like tuna, salmon, swordfish and mackerel, are swimming with omega-3 fatty acids, which have been linked to the prevention of heart disease. A study published in the *Journal of the American Medical Association* suggests that eating one serving of fatty fish per week can reduce the risk of heart attack by up to 70 percent. Those same heart-protecting omega-3s may also provide relief for menstrual cramps, migraine headaches and rheumatoid arthritis as well as help you trim down. In one recent Australian study, overweight men and women who ate a serving of fish rich in omega-3s once a day lowered their cholesterol and lost weight; no such luck for a group of control subjects who ate fish only once a week.

3. Green Tea

No wonder health-conscious people from Los Angeles to Japan are filling up with green tea. Filled with antioxidants that combat free radicals, the soothing brew is believed to stave off various cancers. Research shows it may also help prevent strokes and heart attacks. And it may even help you drop a pound or two. According to a recent study published in the *American Journal of Clinical Nutrition,* green tea drinkers appear to burn calories at an accelerated rate. Don't worry about it interfering with your sleep or dehydrating your skin—green tea is naturally low in caffeine. So plan a good-for-you green tea party!

4. Garlic

Talk about a disease-fighting champion! Garlic has been shown to guard against heart disease by dramatically reducing levels of LDL or "bad" cholesterol and possibly mobilizing fats already deposited in your arteries. Known in past years as "stinking rose," garlic boasts at least 15 different antioxidants, and the National Cancer Institute credits it as a cancer-preventive food. It fights bacteria and gives your immune system a boost.

How much garlic do you need to experience the benefits? There is no general consensus, but some experts say to shoot for at least three cloves a day. You can sneak a lot into pastas, stir-fries, soups and chicken dishes. Or try rubbing a clove on a piece of toast, then top with chopped tomatoes and basil. Sometimes I bake a whole head of garlic, drizzled with a teaspoon of olive oil, and use it instead of butter or margarine on bread.

As far as garlic supplements go, researchers still don't know which components of the clove are potent, and garlic supplements aren't regulated (meaning you have no proof that they're effective), so you're probably better off with the real thing. If you're worried about your breath (I know I am!), try chewing on fresh parsley or a coffee bean after you eat it. I also find it helps to brush and floss right after eating.

5. Blueberries

Filled with antioxidants and unique bacteria-fighting properties, blueberries are an amazing (and tasty) disease-fighting tool. Like cranberries, blueberries may prevent and relieve bladder infections. They contain compounds called anthocyanosides that have been shown to slow down vision loss. And a recent study conducted at the Agriculture Department's Human Nutrition Research Center on Aging at Tufts University in Boston suggests that eating at least a half cup of the blue fruit a day can help improve balance, coordination and short-term memory.

6. Spinach

While you shouldn't expect Popeye's bulging biceps, spinach and other dark leafy greens can provide amazing benefits for your whole body. One cup of cooked spinach contains about 244 milligrams of bone-building calcium—about the same as a cup of milk. It's filled with cancer-fighting beta-carotene and vitamin C; one new study links diets rich in spinach and other dark leafy greens to a significantly lower risk of cancer. Spinach also is loaded with folate, a B vitamin known to help prevent birth defects and thought to protect against heart disease and stroke. And let's not forget fiber: One cup of spinach delivers more than 4 grams.

If you're not a big fan of spinach salad, good news: Research indicates that spinach may be even better for you after it's been lightly sautéed or steamed. Apparently certain antioxidant-like compounds called carotenoids are released during the heating process. But don't overdo it. All it takes is a minute or two to release those carotenoids, and other key vitamins and minerals may be leached out if you overcook. A neat trick I learned from a friend: Buy those bags of prewashed fresh spinach, poke a hole in one side and microwave for a minute. Instant cooked spinach!

7. Flaxseed

Flaxseed contains high amounts of phytoestrogens as well as omega-3 fatty acids, which may help prevent heart disease while keeping your eyes, your brain and your reproductive system healthy. Some studies show flaxseed may even help prevent breast cancer. It also supplies iron, niacin, phosphorus and vitamin E. Like spinach, flaxseed also packs a lot of fiber (about 6 grams per ounce).

To unleash the health benefits of flaxseed, the hard outer coating must be broken down. This can be accomplished by grinding the seeds with a mortar and pestle or popping them in a food processor or pepper mill. Or you can head to your local health food store, where it can be purchased already ground. Like wheat germ, flaxseed's nutty flavor lends itself to baked goods and grain dishes. Try sprinkling it on oatmeal or yogurt, baking it into breads and muffins, or adding it to whole-grain rice or rice pilaf. To make sure it stays fresh, store it in the refrigerator.

8. Oatmeal

Hot or cold, plain or topped with bananas and cinnamon, a hearty bowl of oatmeal can help lower cholesterol—research proves it! Studies show that it can help reduce your level of "bad" LDL cholesterol by as much as 10 percent, earning it the American Heart Association's stamp of approval. This wholesome grain also sticks to your ribs, so you'll have energy for exercise and won't find yourself nibbling an hour later. Try a bowl at breakfast, or bake it into breads, hearty cookies or a refreshing fruit cobbler.

9. Broccoli

Former president George Bush may not like it much, but my family does! I always serve it to my kids with butter and salt, and they think it's great. Broccoli is packed with many unique disease-fighting nutrients. Loaded with antioxidants like beta-carotene and vitamin C, broccoli may help protect against cancer of the colon, lungs and breasts. This fiber-filled veggie can help reduce cholesterol. It also contains lutein, a proven vision saver. Toss chopped raw broccoli into salads, add lightly steamed florets to soups, or stir-fry stalks and sprinkle with toasted sesame seeds.

10. Nuts

For many years we've been told that nuts are a nutritional no-no because they're high in fat and calories. Turns out we were misinformed. When they aren't roasted and salted, nuts are a great preventive tool in the fight against cancer and heart disease. Walnuts and almonds contain antioxidants that help keep arteries healthy while reducing cholesterol. Nuts also contain vitamin E, another important nutrient in the fight against heart disease. Like fish, nuts contain the all-important omega-3 fatty acids. And some varieties of nuts, such as almonds and Brazil nuts, contain selenium, another cancer-fighting mineral that's also good for your skin. Don't worry about blowing your diet: Researchers from Brigham and Women's Hospital in Boston say that nuts satisfy your hunger more than empty snacks like rice cakes or pretzels—so they may actually help you control your eating and your waistline. Just don't go overboard: An ounce of nuts (about a small fistful) or a tablespoon of peanut butter should be enough to deliver a powerful dose of nutrients and curb your appetite. I always keep a small bag of almonds on hand. Saves me from reaching for something unhealthy!

THE 10 AGE ACCELERATORS

Just as there are foods that can help slow the aging process, there are definitely others that help to speed it up. While no food is completely off-limits, you would be wise to watch your intake of these 10 troublemakers:

1. Breakfast "Desserts"

Most donuts, croissants, cinnamon rolls and jumbo muffins are filled with calories and unhealthy fats. They're also devoid of nutrients and lacking in fiber and protein, so you're apt to feel hungry shortly after eating and end up reaching for another high-calorie, non-nutritious nibble like candy. If you can't live without your breakfast sweet, try a toaster muffin (the size of a slice of bread, but it comes in flavors like blueberry and cinnamon) or a small, low-fat bran muffin with a small container of low-fat yogurt or milk (for protein and vitamins) and a piece of fresh fruit (for fiber).

2. Fatty Meats

Nutrition experts have relaxed a bit about the consumption of red meat. Still, you should be aware that roast beef and other fatty meats are rich in artery-sabotaging saturated fat. Several studies show that women who eat meat on a daily basis are 50 percent more likely to suffer heart disease than vegetarian women. Of course, nobody likes a good hamburger more than I do—so I'm not telling you to give it up. I'm merely suggesting that you cut back and opt for lean cuts whenever possible. Choose ground sirloin instead of chuck—it's 90 percent fat-free—or lean steak instead of fatty prime rib. If you're ordering a burger, skip the mayo and special sauces and try mustard or ketchup instead. Your arteries will thank you!

3. Deep-Fried Foods

Just one look at the grease dripping from that pile of french fries and you know that they're naughty. You're right. Deep-fried foods are oozing with saturated and trans fats that have been shown to raise levels of LDL ("bad") cholesterol and increase your heart disease risk. And just think about the way you feel after eating onion rings, beer-battered shrimp and other deep-fried baddies: flabby and sluggish, with no desire to move. If you must have your french fries, try this healthy alternative: Cut russet or sweet potatoes into wedges, then brush with olive oil and dust with herbs and seasonings. Place on a cookie sheet and roast in a preheated 450-degree oven for 30 to 35 minutes.

4. High-Fat Dairy Products

Like red meat, dairy products such as whole milk, cream, butter and full-fat cheese are loaded with calories and fat—the saturated kind that can send cholesterol levels soaring. Again, I'm not asking you to eliminate these foods; just eat them in very small amounts or save them for special occasions. Or do what I do: Lighten your coffee with low-fat or soy milk instead of cream; use low-fat cottage cheese rather than whole-milk ricotta in lasagna; reduce the amount of butter in your recipes (most recipes can actually work with *half* the suggested amount!); and substitute frozen yogurt for whipped cream.

5. Fast Food

With a few exceptions that I talk about on pages 171 and 172, most fast food is a high-fat hazard and nutritional wasteland. One Burger King Whopper has 640 calories and 39 grams of fat—that's over half of your daily fat in one sandwich! Deep-dish pizzas add almost 50 percent more fat than a thin-crust alternative. And then there are the less obvious pitfalls. Chicken salad from Boston Market has as much fat as a super-size order of fries! And a Caesar side salad has more fat than mashed potatoes and gravy. Unless you make friends with the salad bar or order orange juice, don't expect to satisfy any fruit and veggie servings. So beware of the drive-through, or do your homework beforehand so you can make smart choices.

6. Candy

You don't need me to tell you that candy is a nutritional zero. No vitamins, no minerals, no benefits for your body whatsoever—only tons of sugar and calories. A few candy corns or Hershey's Kisses certainly won't kill you, but think twice about raiding that candy dish or box of chocolates on a regular basis. There are many more nutritious ways to satisfy that sugar craving—dried fruit, seedless grapes, strawberries or a frozen banana, to name a few.

7. Processed Lunch Meats

Most hot dogs, sausages and processed meats like bologna are filled with color and flavor enhancers like sodium nitrite and nitrate. When heated, these preservatives form highly carcinogenic (cancer-causing) compounds called nitrosamines. If you're at a ballpark or backyard BBQ, you'd be better off with a piece of grilled chicken (skinless) or even a hamburger. At home, I heat up a tofu or soy dog—they're actually quite good and free of nitrites.

8. Creamy Salad Dressings

I used to be a big salad person—I loved the idea of sitting down to a heaping bowl of food without feeling guilty. Salad was the ultimate healthy food! Then came my reality check. Turns out a salad drenched in creamy or oily dressing may have more calories and fat than a burger and fries. Thousand Island dressing delivers approximately 260 calories and 26 grams of fat per ¼ cup. Some honey French dressings weigh in at 280 calories and 23 grams of fat. A typical serving of blue cheese dressing runs around 160 calories and 16 fat grams. And since many restaurant salads come dripping with dressing, chances are you're getting much more than a single serving. Best bets: Ask for your dressing on the side and pick a low-fat vinaigrette or balsamic dressing. Ordering a salad is great—just make sure yours isn't dressed to kill.

9. Stick Margarine

Once considered a healthy alternative to butter, researchers now say that stick margarine may be just as bad for your arteries. Margarine is formed when vegetable oils are hydrogenated to create a firm texture. During the hydrogenation process, the heart-healthy oils turn into trans fats, which have been shown to raise LDL, or "bad," cholesterol. Soft, tub margarine contains fewer trans fats than margarine that comes in a stick.

Some people like the taste of margarine. Personally, I prefer butter—and since I found out about trans fats, I've chosen to use small amounts of the real stuff on my English muffin or sweet potato. On toast, I try to use low-sugar fruit spreads or a cholesterol-lowering spread like Take Control, which doesn't taste as good as butter but isn't bad. When I cook, I always opt for heart-healthy olive oil over butter or margarine.

10. Greasy Snack Chips

While they may come from healthy sources like potatoes and corn, packaged snack chips are filled with fat and calories—and, sadly, little or no nutritional value. And as the saying goes, "Nobody can eat just one." To top it off, they're often vehicles for high-fat dips and spreads. If you're in the mood for some mindless munching, reach for carrots (buy the already peeled and washed kind) or air-popped popcorn (filled with fiber). If it's salt that you're craving, try pretzels or baked tortilla chips (much lower in fat but very tasty) with a little salsa. If you must have your Doritos, buy a small single-serving package—but not every day if you can help it!

MAKING IT WORK

Eat more often. Load up on leafy greens. Trade your bagel for a bowl of bran flakes. Start every meal with soup. It all makes perfect sense on paper, but how do you make it a reality for you and your family? Breaking old habits is hard enough, much less adopting new ones. But you can do it—and once you do, you'll realize how satisfying and delicious healthy eating can be.

Don't try to overhaul your eating habits all in one day. That's a recipe for failure! Start by choosing four specific nutrition goals that seem doable—for example, upping your intake of fruits and veggies; drinking 8 to 10 glasses of water a day; taking a multivitamin; and introducing soy into your diet. You'll find a place to record your goals on page 244.

Over the next four weeks we'll be working on these four goals one at a time. For example: During Week 1, you'll focus on Goal No. 1. During Week 2, you'll also work on Goal No. 2. During Week 3, your priority will be Goal No. 3. And so on. At the end of the month, you'll have four wonderful new habits that I want you to continue practicing. It might be a while before you do all these things instinctively, without thinking about them—but I promise you that day will come. You'll also identify and begin tackling your next four healthy eating goals.

Even if you're an experienced cook, one of your big challenges may be introducing anti-aging foods like flaxseed into your diet. To make the task easier, I've featured these nutritional powerhouses in the healthy recipes later on in the book. (You'll even find one that calls for cancer-fighting green tea!) Or you can reinvent some of your family favorites—a few years ago, for instance, I started adding crumbled soy protein to my pasta sauces. My girls never even tasted the difference!

On the following pages, you'll find other helpful hints for slashing the fat, adding more variety to your diet and making smart choices when it comes to fast food and take-out. There *will* be occasions when you simply don't have time to prepare a healthy meal. Don't worry: It happens to me all the time! Fortunately, I've figured out ways to turn a deli sandwich or even a frozen pizza into a nutritious meal. Here's your opportunity to really get creative.

A Return to Healthy Home Cooking

My mother was a wonderful cook. Growing up, she used to wow the family with rich foods like macaroni and cheese, mashed potatoes and chocolate cheesecake. But a few years ago, during a visit to her California home, I cracked down on her "comfort foods." While her gooey lasagnas and buttery blueberry muffins were positively mouthwatering, I was worried about her health as well as my dad's.

Studies from Harvard Medical School and other top research facilities continue to show that a diet low in saturated fat is crucial for a healthy heart. Fortunately, minimizing your intake of this artery-damaging fat doesn't have to mean giving up meat or cutting out oil and butter altogether. Your food doesn't have to taste like cardboard, either, and I offer tips for turning low-fat meals into satisfying treats later in this section. First, I'd like to share the three golden rules that form my healthy-cooking bible.

Rule No. 1: Think Lean As I've said before, you need a little fat in your diet. The key is to choose your fats wisely. By that I mean mainly sticking to lean meats like chicken and turkey, fish (including shellfish) and low-fat dairy products. Olive and canola oils, avocados and nuts are also healthy choices; the fat they contain is unsaturated, meaning it won't harm your arteries.

For me, the easiest way to distinguish the "good" fat from "bad" fat is to focus on the source. If the fat is from plants or the sea, it's a good choice; if it's from animals, it could be trouble. This isn't science—it's simply my rule of thumb.

These days you can buy cuts of meat or ground meat—including beef, pork, turkey and chicken—that are up to 98 or 99 percent fat free.

If you're cooking chicken, opt for skinless or remove the fatty skin before putting it in the oven. Chicken and turkey sausage are better alternatives to beef or pork.

Let's not forget: No food is off-limits—and that even goes for juicy prime rib, succulent sausage and crispy bacon. Even I like to sink my teeth into a burger or a BLT occasionally! Just try not to make it a habit. Believe it or not, once you go from fatty to lean, you may actually lose your taste for rich foods like roast beef—really!

Fats: The Good, the Bad and the Ugly

Not all fats are created equal—some offer benefits while others can be harmful. Here's how to tell the difference:

Monounsaturated
What it is: This good fat raises your HDL, or "good," cholesterol and therefore may help protect against heart disease. Monounsaturated fat is liquid at room temperature but starts to solidify when refrigerated.
Where you'll find it: Avocados, cashews, olives, peanuts, olive oil, peanut oil, peanut butter, canola oil.

Polyunsaturated
What it is: Like monounsaturated fats, these heart-healthy fats may help reduce heart disease risk. Polyunsaturated fats stay in liquid form whether cold or at room temperature.
Where you'll find it: Almonds, walnuts, pecans, fish, safflower oil, soybean oil, sunflower oil, corn oil

Saturated
What it is: Saturated fat raises your LDL, or "bad," cholesterol and contributes to heart disease and other health problems. Less than 10 percent of your total daily calories should come from saturated fat. This fat "devil" remains solid at any temperature. For example, think of the fat that you find around the edge of a cut of beef.
Where you'll find it: Butter, cheese, chocolate, coconut and coconut oil, egg yolks, lard, meat, whole milk, palm oil

Trans
What it is: Trans fats start off as heart-healthy vegetable oil (olive, canola, corn, etc.), but when the oil is hydrogenated to make it solid, it undergoes a chemical process that turns it into a bad fat. Recent research shows that trans fats act a lot like saturated fats, increasing your LDL cholesterol levels and your risk of heart disease.
Where you'll find it: French fries, onion rings, donuts, stick margarine, cinnamon rolls, cheese Danish, microwave popcorn, buttermilk biscuits, vegetable shortening

Rule No. 2: Strive for Balance About 10 years ago I used to sit down to a giant (and I mean huge!) bowl of pasta with steamed veggies and fat-free spaghetti sauce for dinner. Afterward I'd feel full but not really satisfied. Soon, I'd find myself searching for that little extra "something"—a piece of bread, ice cream, a chunk of chocolate.

Back then, pasta was considered the ultimate diet food, yet I wasn't as lean as I am now. As it turns out, I was going a little overboard on the carbo loading. Without a healthy balance of carbohydrates (about 50 to 55 percent of total calories), protein (about 20 to 25 percent of total calories) and fat (25 percent of total calories)—ideally with each meal—you won't be able to cover your nutritional bases, and as a result, your body won't feel as satisfied. That's when the urge to snack kicks in.

Today, instead of only pasta and vegetables (pure carbohydrate), I'll

Color-Me-Healthy Grocery Guide

Reds
Tomatoes, tomato juice or sauce, red peppers, beets, radishes, raspberries, strawberries, apples, red grapes, watermelon, cranberries, cranberry juice, pomegrantes, ruby-red grapefruit, cherries, red potatoes, red onions, kidney beans

Oranges
Carrots, sweet potatoes, pumpkins, acorn or butternut squash, orange peppers, cantaloupe, tangerines, peaches, mangos, papayas, apricots

Yellows
Squash, corn, sweet yellow peppers, onions, bananas, pineapples, lemons, pears, grapefruit, turnips

Greens
Spinach, broccoli, zucchini, asparagus, green peppers, lima beans, peas, Brussels sprouts, romaine or green-leaf lettuce, kale, beet or collard greens, leeks, green beans, cucumbers, celery, avocados, green onions, edamame, fresh herbs, kiwi fruit, limes, honeydew melon, green grapes, Granny Smith apples, star fruit

Blues/Purples
Eggplant, blueberries, purple grapes, blackberries, plums, raisins, purple potatoes, purple peppers, black beans

Browns
Whole-grain cereal, oat bran, brown rice, wheat germ, flaxseed, lentils, garbanzo beans, russet potatoes, nuts, sunflower seeds, mushrooms, figs

White
Cauliflower, endive, onions, parsnips, fennel

Healthy Kitchen Makeover

Over the years, we've constantly reinvented ourselves—and now it's time to reinvent your kitchen to suit your new, healthier lifestyle.

Purge your pantry. Get rid of old-fashioned, unhealthy items to make room for newer, lighter ones. High-fat salad dressings are a thing of the past; try a low-fat raspberry vinaigrette or balsamic vinegar. Creamy soups can go—trade them for vegetable or bean soups that are lower in fat and salt. Swap real sour cream and mayo for reduced-fat sour cream and Dijon mustard. Push aside the palm and coconut oil to make way for heart-healthy olive or canola oil. Replace stick margarine with tub margarine (lower in unhealthy trans fats). Ditch the chocolates, fudge cookies and tub of toffee crunch ice cream. Why tempt yourself?

Stock up on healthy snacks. Keeping plenty of nutritious nibbles at home and work will help you avoid trips to the cookie jar or vending machine. Fresh fruit, carrots, celery, whole-wheat crackers and air-popped popcorn provide fiber and complex carbohydrates. Sliced turkey breast, reduced-fat cheese, hummus, natural peanut butter, soy nuts, and low-fat yogurt are quick sources of protein. To satisfy a sweet tooth, try dried fruit, graham crackers, Fig Newtons, ginger cookies, frozen fudge pops, frozen yogurt bars, and sorbet.

Spruce up your spice rack. Seductive flavors like curry, cumin, cinnamon, allspice and vanilla will add zest to low-fat entrées and desserts. And with fresh ground pepper, red pepper flakes and Tabasco, who needs the saltshaker?

Invest in a Steamer or a Wok. Steaming and stir-frying are two of the healthiest ways to cook. If you don't have a steamer, a wok or a nonstick skillet, consider buying one. You'll be making a deposit in your good-health IRA!

sauté diced chicken (protein) and veggies (carbohydrate) in a little olive oil (fat), then top it with tomato sauce. I skip the pasta altogether. For me, it's the perfect, feel-good meal. Every time I eat it—or a similar combo—I feel completely content and energized.

Rule No. 3: Mix It Up Eating the same foods all the time isn't just boring—it gyps your body of nutrients needed to prevent the ravages of aging. Research shows that people who eat a wide variety of foods live longer than those who constantly eat the same old things. Since it's easy to get stuck in a rut or gravitate to old favorites, you may want to try this simple mix-it-up strategy: Fill your grocery cart with reds, oranges, yellows, greens, blues and browns. The more hues, the better! Then paint your plates with a rainbow of color. Serve grilled fish with a red pepper, carrot and zucchini medley. Broiled chicken goes beautifully with mashed sweet potatoes and asparagus spears. Drop blueberries, raspberries and kiwi on your breakfast cereal. Each meal should look like a painting by Picasso or Matisse!

Satisfy Your Senses: How to Give Life to Low-Fat Food

Bland, boring, dull, disappointing—these are the words that may come to mind when we talk about healthy cooking. But low-fat food doesn't have to be ho-hum, uninspired and flavorless. In fact it can be just the opposite, especially if you focus on satisfying the senses of taste, sight, touch and smell. Here are four delicious ways to add zip to low-fat dishes and lite bites:

1. Do yourself a flavor. After years of "Mom" food, low-fat cuisine may sound about as appetizing as cardboard. True, fat brings out the flavor in food, so some meals might taste a little bland without it. The answer isn't adding a lot of salt or extra oil. You can enhance the taste of your food by using lots of fresh herbs and powerful spices. Thai and Indian flavors such as curry and cumin pep up soups and chicken dishes. Cinnamon, nutmeg, allspice and vanilla add a sweet touch to oatmeal and applesauce. Fresh herbs like oregano, tarragon, thyme and sage bring a new dimension to pasta sauces, lasagna

Food Face-lifts

A few little changes can make a big nutritional difference in your day. So try giving some of your old favorites the following 21st-century twists:

Instead of	Choose
Stick margarine	Tub margarine
Plain bagel	A whole-grain bagel
Pasta	Whole-wheat pasta
Chicken fingers	Chicken satay
Chinese food	Sushi
Peanut butter	Natural peanut butter or soy butter
Iceberg lettuce	Spinach
Croutons	Roasted soy nuts
Cream cheese	Low-fat cream cheese or tofu spread
Hot dog	Soy dog
Hamburger	Turkey or veggie burger
Sausage	Spicy chicken sausage
Jelly beans	Dried apples, pears or cranberries
Frozen yogurt	Nonfat chai tea latte
Cola	Seltzer with a splash of cranberry juice

and egg-white omelets. Fresh basil with sliced tomatoes and a drizzle of olive oil or balsamic vinegar is heavenly.

2. Give it eye appeal. Whether you're preparing food for a dinner party or for one, presentation counts almost as much as taste. Resist the urge to eat a frozen entrée straight from the container or stuff in a sandwich while standing over the kitchen sink. It only takes a few minutes to create a visual feast. A simple sprig of basil or a slice of lemon can give food a gourmet feel. Or try painting your plate with the most colorful foods possible—it will please your eyes *and* provide a wide range of nutrients.

3. Sink your teeth into it. To keep my mouth interested and my tummy content, I think of the four Cs—chewy, crunchy, crispy and creamy. Team crunchy cereal with smooth yogurt and chewy raisins. Try chewy spinach salad with crunchy toasted walnuts and cool pears. Top crispy wheat crackers with creamy soy butter. Every bite will be a satisfying surprise!

4. Be scent-sible. Lemon zest. Peppermint tea. Freshly baked bread. Roasted garlic. Who ever said low-fat food was blah? Whether you're warming up with a cup of chai tea or eating a tangerine, take a moment to indulge in the scent. Your nose will send a "delicious treat ahead" signal to your tummy.

Timesaving Strategies

My life is pretty hectic sometimes, with two kids, a husband, and a full-time job. Finding time to prepare my own meals is a challenge—but I make a point of it because it's the best way to ensure good nutrition for the entire family. I like to know what's going into each dish! To make it more doable, I've learned to minimize time spent at the supermarket, streamline preparation and cut down on cleanup. Here are four approaches that work for the Austin family, and they'll work for yours.

Plan your meals for the week. Every Monday, I try to sit down with a pad of paper and outline meals for the next seven days. I usually plan a few meals that make good leftovers (a hearty soup, veggie lasagna or chicken casserole) or can be disguised as brand-new dishes—Sunday's roast turkey turns into Monday's turkey sandwiches, Tuesday's turkey soup and Wednesday's low-fat turkey pot pie.

Do grocery shopping during off-peak hours. I'm lucky, because my schedule is flexible, to have time during the week to shop. (I avoid doing it on the weekends.) Since I've already mapped out my meals for the week, I bring a detailed list so I don't forget anything. (They say the memory is the first thing to go!) Missing a key ingredient while rushing to get dinner ready can really blow your cool.

Many cities have grocery delivery services. Check out the Internet, as my sister in California did. She now orders everything online!

Get cooking! Prepare as much healthy food ahead of time as you can. Chop up veggies and store in a Tupperware container for quick snacks and last-minute salads. In a tightly sealed container, fruit salad will last a few days; toss chunks on top of your breakfast cereal or serve with yogurt for dessert.

Keep it simple. I love to experiment with new recipes, but during the week I stick to the basics—recipes my family loves that have just a few ingredients and which I know by heart (see my Tricky Quickies, below). Save the fancy stuff for weekends or special occasions!

Make it a group effort. My girls love to help toss the salad or set the table, and Jeff often takes care of the cleanup. Don't be afraid to ask your husband and kids to help out—they probably won't volunteer. It's fun to have company, and you can cut kitchen time in half! Meals should not become your responsibility alone.

Denise's Tricky Quickies

On busy weekday nights I like to make my Tricky Quickies—speedy meals that don't require a lot of preparation or cleanup. For example, the "All-in-One-Oven" dinner: Just preheat the oven to 350 degrees. Baking potatoes go in first. Thirty minutes later I place chicken breasts on a disposable broiler pan and put them in the oven, too. After 15 more minutes I add asparagus spears wrapped in aluminum foil and tightly sealed so they "steam." Total cooking time: one hour for the potato; 30 minutes for the chicken; 15 minutes for the asparagus. An almost-elegant meal with no pots!

Another quick family favorite is Girl Scout Hash. (I learned this one on a camping trip.) Boil rotini (spiral pasta), rinse, drain, stir in 1 tablespoon olive oil, and set aside. In the same pot, brown chopped onion and lean ground beef or turkey. Add chunky vegetable tomato sauce and heat. Just before serving, dump in the pasta! Toss in some baby spinach leaves for a hearty, well-rounded meal with only one pot to clean.

Don't forget the Tricky Quickies that you can create with leftovers. Cook double amounts of meat and rice one night, then reheat the next night with a change of veggies and a different sauce. You'll find more fast-and-easy weeknight meal ideas in the recipe section.

Take-out: A Healthy Twist

You're constantly juggling a million different things. Maybe you have a husband, kids or aging parents to care for. Or maybe your 9-to-5 job is more like 9-to-9. In between, there's housework, chauffeuring, shopping and workouts. You'd love to cook beautiful meals—but when?

For many women with overloaded schedules, take-out isn't just a convenience, it's a lifesaver. Sadly, store-bought meals can really wreak havoc on your waistline. The problems include monster portion sizes that are high in fat and calories as well as meals that are deficient in fruits and veggies.

Fortunately, there are ways to up the nutrient profile of your take-out meal—if you know what to do and what to watch for. These dos and don'ts can help you maximize your nutrients while avoiding those pesky dieting pitfalls.

The Deli
DON'T

- Think tuna, chicken and egg salad are a good choice—unless the deli uses low-fat mayonnaise.
- Accept the chips, fries or pasta salad side dish that might be offered. Ask for cottage cheese instead.
- Order cream soups—go for veggie- or broth-based soups.

DO

- Opt for whole-grain, whole-wheat or pumpernickel bread over white, sourdough or rye.
- Request mustard instead of mayo.
- Choose turkey, lean roast beef or ham without cheese.
- Ask for lettuce or spinach, tomato, cucumber and sprouts, if available.
- Ask for less. I'll often order a sandwich with half the meat or just one slice of cheese. Don't be afraid to speak up to get exactly what you and your healthy body want.

The Drive-Through
DON'T

- Go to fast-food restaurants expecting a large choice for a woman over 40. There are very few healthy options.
- Go when you're hungry—you'll order fries.
- "Super-size" or "combo" anything. Women over 40 do not need any substance named "jumbo."

DO

- Check out the salad dressings before using—choose low-calorie options if available.
- Go grill, girl! If there is a grilled fish or chicken item, it's your best bet.
- Substitute veggies for fries or onion rings whenever possible.
- Sit down to eat. Wolfing down a hamburger while you drive is *less* satisfying than taking 10 minutes to enjoy a fresh salad.

The Pizza Parlor

DON'T

- Get any fatty extras. Skip the extra cheese, pepperoni and sausage.
- Order deep-dish. Super-rich, fatty and heavy, these pies toss in high numbers for both calories and fat.

DO

- Order a whole-wheat crust—it's extra fiber and extra flavor!
- Load up on veggies—try broccoli, fresh tomatoes or my favorite, spinach and garlic.

Take It Out, Bring It Home

Who said homemade food has to be cooked all at home? I like doing "combo" meals—that is, meals that are part take-out and part prepared by me. It's quick and easy, yet I still have control over what my family is eating. Here, a few nutritious examples:

- Add spinach leaves to soups or deli sandwiches.

- Make a stir-fry using precut veggies from the supermarket salad bar and frozen shrimp.

- Lightly steam or sauté salad bar veggies and add to soups, pasta sauces or frozen dinners.

- Top bakery-made angel food cake with fresh or thawed frozen fruit—elegant yet easy.

- Add leftover chicken to a store-bought pasta-and-veggie salad. Eat it cold or warm!

- Accompany a frozen, low-fat veggie lasagna (another Austin family favorite) with a nutritious side salad. I pop the lasagna in the oven, stretch for 20 minutes, then chop those veggies. There's even time to cut up some fresh fruit for dessert!

- Try part-skim ricotta on your pizza instead of mozzarella—it's a new taste and a great source of calcium.
- Go for the thin crust—the thinner, the better.

The Supermarket

While we tend to think of supermarkets as places to buy produce and other staples, they also provide a lot of quick picks ranging from frozen entrées to fresh salads.

Frozen Dinners

DON'T

- Expect a lot of veggies in these frozen meals. My solution: Lightly steam chopped veggies like snow peas, carrots and zucchini—almost anything goes—and toss them on top. Or fix a small green salad—with low-cal dressing, of course.
- Forget to read the labels. Many frozen entrées look healthy, but check the label for fat and calories. You may be surprised by what you find!

DO

- Try light frozen entrées from companies like Weight Watchers, Lean Cuisine and Healthy Choice—they have their perks. They are the perfect size—not too big or too small. The calories and fat are shown on the label. They're ready in minutes. And many of them are truly quite tasty.
- Experiment! Use these prepackaged items as a base for your own spices and kitchen creativity. You'll add zing to a quick fix.

Pre-Roasted Meats

These days, take-out is so popular that many supermarkets offer an inviting array of pre-roasted, ready-to-eat chickens and turkeys. These are great, healthy, low-fat dinner options when you're pressed for time. (Just take the skin off.) I'll pick one up along with some quick-cook brown rice and broccoli and whip together a wholesome, "home-cooked" meal in 15 minutes. The chickens and turkeys are kept under a heat lamp at the store, so you don't even need to heat them. In most markets you can also find precooked, presliced poultry from companies like Perdue. Microwave some veggies and a potato to go with your bird, or cut into cubes and toss into pasta, soups and salads.

Salad Bars

DON'T

- Take anything loaded with mayonnaise.
- Pile on the croutons or bacon bits. If you want a crunchy topping, try a sprinkle of sunflower seeds.
- Ladle on cream-based dressings (ranch, Caesar, creamy Italian or French). If it doesn't say "low-fat," watch out!

DO

- Opt for spinach over iceberg lettuce, since darker greens are more nutrient-packed.
- Load up on veggies—chopped broccoli, carrots, tomatoes, peppers or sprouts.
- Add protein by sprinkling on tuna (without mayo), kidney beans or crumbled low-fat cheese—feta or goat cheese, for example.
- Go for the low-fat or vinaigrette dressings.
- Include a side of fresh fruit for dessert.

The Gourmet Shop

If it's like mine, your local gourmet shop—you know, the one with 10 exotic brands of olive oil and imported coffee—is full of mouthwatering meals and salads. The trick is to find the healthy alternatives mixed in with the high-fat foods.

DON'T

- Order anything filled or topped with cheeses or made with cream, butter or sour cream.
- Try anything that is fried or breaded.
- Give in to temptation! Gourmet shops make everything look wonderful and delicious—and no doubt it is—but you'll feel better if you stick with the healthy alternatives that are hiding behind the alfredo sauce.
- Look too longingly at the cookie or dessert display at your local take-out place. Instead of giving in, substitute a fat-free chocolate mint instead. Your sweet tooth will be satisfied and your waistline stays intact.

DO

- Look for grilled or steamed options (fish, chicken, tofu).
- Take control. You pay by the pound, so if you want only 4 ounces of chicken, make sure that's what you get. Remember, the customer is always right.
- Load up on veggies. Try grilled or roasted veggies (zucchini,

mushrooms, peppers—just pass on the eggplant since it soaks up a lot of oil). Look for steamed veggies or a mixed veggie salad.

- Be exotic! Try new and different fruits and veggies that are being showcased. You may find a new favorite like star fruit, guava or pomegranate. And for me, there is no bigger treat than slices of fresh mango.

Once you learn how to pick healthier items from your grocery store and add home food for a good, nutritional balance, you can do take-out with a good conscience and taste-tempting flair. Now, go out there and order well—you can do it!

Keep a Food Diary

Fast-food courts. Vending machines. Jumbo-sized portions. As much as you'd like to eat well, it isn't always easy—especially when you're surrounded by temptation. While you shouldn't feel guilty for occasionally caving in to a Big Mac or ice cream sundae, you don't want to do it all the time, especially if you're watching your waistline. As I mentioned before, you also need to save room for nutritious foods that will help give you gorgeous skin and hair and defend your body against illness.

Whether you're trying to drop weight or just get healthy, research shows that a food diary can help you avoid empty calories—especially during the holidays and other high-risk situations like business dinners and weddings. Start by buying a notebook, then record what you eat for breakfast, lunch and dinner in addition to between-meal nibbles. Try to include portion sizes so you can get an accurate gauge on your food intake. And don't forget to include things like breath mints and chewing gum. You may be surprised at how many useless "extras" you're actually eating.

While a little snacking is healthy, the calories can really add up if you don't watch it. Here's a perfect example: One tablespoon of peanut butter, a handful of chips and a chocolate-covered cherry from that heart-shaped box come out to about 200 calories. Consume an extra 200 calories per day without changing your exercise habits, and you can put on almost *10* pounds in six months.

Common Diet Dilemmas

Diet Dilemma No. 1

Problem: "Every time I go to a wedding or fund-raiser, I end up eating whatever is placed in front of me—usually something much too big and very fattening."

Solution: We've all been there—faced with a four-course meal that includes salad dripping with oil, a giant slab of fatty meat, an endless supply of dinner rolls and a gooey dessert. What to do? Try speaking with your server. Today many banquet halls and restaurants keep a few vegetarian meals on hand. If not, don't feel obligated to clean your plate, and watch out for side dishes like creamed spinach and potatoes au gratin. As for the dinner rolls, try to avoid them, or stick to hearty, whole-grain choices and breadsticks rather than white, French or foccacia. To prevent the dessert temptation, take a pass before the dish is placed in front of you or ask for a healthier alternative such as fresh fruit or sorbet. A cappuccino made with skim milk also may satisfy your urge for sweets. Most important, be sure to eat a healthy, fiber-rich snack such as an apple or whole-wheat crackers topped with reduced-fat peanut butter *before* your event; definitely don't show up hungry. Or fill up on healthy veggies during the cocktail hour. Remember—the best defense is a good offense!

Diet Dilemma No. 2

Problem: "My job requires a lot of traveling and eating out at restaurants with business associates and clients."

Solution: Restaurants today are working hard to provide at least a few healthy options. Broiled fish may not sound as enticing as the pasta carbonara that your business colleague ordered, but trust me—you'll be happier in the long run. If you don't find a suitable option on the menu, don't be embarrassed to ask. Many kitchens are willing to put together a plate of healthy basics like broiled or grilled chicken, a baked potato and steamed veggies. Or try to mix and match from the healthier-sounding options on the menu. Ask about portion size before placing your order. If portions tend to be large, request a half portion, or stick to soup and a small appetizer or green salad. When I'm on the road (which is often!), I try to eat a big lunch and keep dinner small. For lunch, I may order salmon with wild rice and vegetables, plus a small green salad. Dinner would be a piece of grilled chicken, soup or a baked potato.

Diet Dilemma No. 3

Problem: "The holidays are always my downfall—every year I pig out on sweets and gain at least five pounds."

Solution: Parties, rich desserts, candy dishes everywhere—as we all know, the holidays can wreak havoc on your waistline. Can you successfully avoid the annual overeat-a-thon? Absolutely. It just takes a little willpower and some careful planning. One of the best ways to forgo those fattening nibbles is to fill yourself up with wholesome foods at breakfast and lunch. Really focus on getting those five to eight servings of fruits and veggies, drinking lots of water and consuming foods rich in fiber. (I suggest making a list of daily goals to keep yourself on track.) If you eat healthy during the first part of the day, you'll probably want to continue nourishing your body with nutrient-dense foods. If you're going to a party, make sure you don't arrive hungry. Have a healthy, fiber-filled snack or maybe even a frozen dinner beforehand. After you arrive, drink lots of water and seltzer to fill yourself up. If you still have the munchies, park yourself near the chopped veggies and away from the desserts. Your hostess is pushing her homemade fudge brownies? If you *really* want one, go ahead—you can compensate by exercising a little longer the following day. If you can live without it, say something like, "I know how addictive your brownies are, and if I have one, I may just eat the whole plate." Remind yourself that nothing tastes as good as feeling good feels. Appease your sweet tooth by chewing a stick of sugarless gum or sucking on a mint. And watch the alcoholic beverages. Those eggnogs and punches not only deliver a lot of calories, they're apt to undermine your resolve to eat healthy.

Diet Dilemma No. 4

Problem: "My healthy eating habits often go down the tubes when I'm around my friends, my husband or my kids."

Solution: They don't mean to do it, but they always seem to open a bag of chips, order a pizza, or bake a fabulous-looking chocolate cheesecake whenever you're having a weak moment. What's a woman over 40 to do? We simply cannot eat the way our husbands and children do. Tell your loved ones about your desire to revamp your eating habits or lose weight, and ask them to stop tempting you with fatty foods and nutritional zeroes. You're not asking *them* to stop eating, of course—just to refrain from sharing and to remind you of your goals when you reach for the potato chip bag. Another alternative is to fight back—instead of chips, break out the air-popped popcorn. Rather than chocolate cheesecake, offer to bring a less sinful dessert like angel food cake topped with yogurt and fresh berries. If you know your girlfriends want to order pizza, come armed with an alternative—a frozen dinner, a homemade salad or a turkey sandwich. And if you have to, turn down invitations involving food. Instead of a lunch date, how about a walking date? Meet for a game of tennis or a bike ride instead of at the local café for coffee and a sweet. Turning back the clock requires strategy and thought—so just keep thinking!

Diet Dilemma No. 5

Problem: "I'm in the car or at the mall, starving for a light lunch to tide me over, and all I see are fast-food restaurants. There goes my diet!"

Solution: Believe it or not, most fast food restaurants *do* have choices compatible with a healthy diet. Take Burger King, for instance. The broiled chicken salad with 200 calories and 10 fat grams (before dressing) is one great option. Next, opt for chicken tenders (310 calories and 17 grams of fat). Even a plain hamburger at 330 calories and 15 grams of fat isn't bad. Also, a 300-calorie vanilla shake (with 6 fat grams) would do in a pinch.

If you pull up at McDonald's, try the plain hamburger (260 calories and 9 fat grams), the Grilled Chicken Salad Deluxe (120 calories and 1.5 fat grams) or the Grilled Chicken Deluxe sandwich (440 calories and 20 fat grams). At 290 calories and 17 fat grams, the 6-piece Chicken McNuggets are another good choice. Likewise, Hardee's offers a 270-calorie burger (11 fat grams), grilled chicken sandwich (350 calories and 11 fat grams) or grilled chicken salad (150 calories and 3 fat grams).

When you see a Subway sign, slow down. They have a Veggie Delite sandwich on whole-wheat bread at 237 calories and 3 fat grams, and turkey on whole-wheat bread at 289 calories and 4 grams of fat—both good choices nutritionally. Wendy's also caters to the diet-conscious with a Garden Veggie Pita (400 calories and 17 grams of fat), grilled chicken sandwich (290 calories and 7 fat grams) and a wide range of salad choices.

If it's breakfast you're missing, Hardee's offers an Apple Cinnamon 'N' Raisin Biscuit (200 calories and 8 fat grams) or pancakes (280 calories and 2 fat grams), or you can pair an Apple Cinnamon 'N' Raisin Biscuit (200 calories and 8 fat grams) with orange juice (140 calories and 0 fat grams). McDonald's has scrambled eggs (160 calories and 11 grams fat), hotcakes (310 calories and 7 grams of fat) or a low-fat apple bran muffin (300 calories and 3 grams fat). Even an Egg McMuffin (290 calories and 12 grams fat) is a decent option.

YOUR 28-DAY CHALLENGE

Once again, it's time to write down your specific nutrition goals for the next weeks. These are just a few suggestions. Remember, you don't have to accomplish everything at once. This is not a diet. It's a plan for the rest of your life.

Week 1: Vow to drink your eight glasses of water each day
Week 2: Cut out fried foods
Week 3: Strive for five; make sure you get five veggies or fruits a day
Week 4: Reduce salt and sugar and include soy

At the end of 28 days, you should have four healthy new habits, ones that will serve you well in the coming years.

THE TURN BACK THE CLOCK MEAL PLAN

To make healthy eating easier for you, I asked nutritionist Leslie Bonci, R.D., to create a 7-day meal plan that includes three meals and two snacks per day. This easy, low-fat eating plan features top anti-aging foods like soy, fish and flaxseed and provides an ideal balance of protein, carbohydrates and healthy fats. Each daily menu also delivers approximately five to seven servings of antioxidant-rich fruits and vegetables, 1,000 to 1,200 milligrams of bone-building calcium and 25 to 30 grams of cancer-fighting fiber. I hope this meal plan will give you some ideas of how to successfully incorporate all of the dietary strategies we've discussed into your daily life.

This 1,800-calorie-per-day plan is designed for active women who want to lose weight gradually and safely. For those of you who are more sedentary or have more pounds to lose, I've also provided a 1,600-calorie-per-day option. Unless you have special circumstances that warrant it, I don't recommend dropping below 1,600 calories per day. If you're exercising (which you should be!), 1,600 is really the minimum number of calories you need to keep your body running in peak condition and to provide the vitamins and nutrients you need.

If there are foods that you dislike or can't eat due to allergies, feel free to substitute one meal for another or modify recipes slightly. I've included extra recipes in the appendix at the end of this book. But do try to maintain a similar calorie count and balance of foods. In other words, don't drop the apple and add an ice cream cone. Use your head!

Shopping List

My Turn Back the Clock 7-day meal plan is designed for one person. If you're cooking for a family, simply multiply the quantities in the shopping list and recipes accordingly. Many of the ingredients listed below come in packages that are larger than what is needed for the 7-day plan—and you may want to make several servings anyway, regardless of the number of mouths you have to feed. Leftovers can be a great incentive to continue your healthy eating habits in the weeks to come. Consider it an investment toward your new, healthy pantry and lighter, younger, livelier lifestyle!

Staples

Oatmeal—1 canister quick-cooking oats (about 18 oz)

Cinnamon

Salsa—1 small jar, any type

Multi-Grain Cheerios—1 small box (about 11.5 oz)

Almonds—1 small package (about 2.5 oz)

Walnuts—1 small package (about 2.3 oz)

Olive oil—1 small bottle (about 17 oz)

Minced garlic—1 small jar

Minced or grated ginger—1 small jar (about 4 oz)

Brown rice—1 small package

Chunky natural peanut butter—1 small jar (about 12 oz)

Golden raisins—1 small box

Dried apricots—5 apricots or 1 small package

Craisins—1 small package (sweetened, dried cranberries made by Ocean Spray—you can find them near the raisins in the food store)

Prunes—5 prunes or 1 small package

Couscous—1 small box (about 10 oz)

Pizza sauce—1 small jar (about 14 oz)

Tomato sauce—1 small jar (about 26 oz) (I like Healthy Choice)

Brown sugar—1 small box

Tuna—1 small can, water-packed (about 3 oz)

Salmon—1 small can (about 7.5 oz)

Light mayonnaise—1 small jar

Low-fat cinnamon or honey oat granola bars—1 small box (about 10 bars)

Mandarin oranges—1 small can (about 6 oz)

Pasta—1 small package, any type (about 16 oz)

Jumbo pasta shells—1 small box (about 12 oz)

Light syrup—1 small bottle (about 12 oz)

Spicy stewed tomatoes—1 small can (about 14.5 oz)

Fat-free bean dip—1 small container or can (about 9 oz)

Frozen Foods

Soy (or veggie) burgers/patties—1 package of 4

Spinach—1 small box (about 10 oz)

Whole-grain waffles—1 small box

Perishables

Dairy

Skim milk—1 half gallon
Orange juice—1 quart
Vanilla yogurt—3 8-oz containers
Lemon yogurt—1 8-oz container
Light cheddar cheese—1 small
    package, shredded (about 8 oz)
Light cheddar cheese—1 small
    package, sliced (about 12 oz)

Part-skim mozzarella cheese—1
    8-oz package
Whipped butter—1 small con-
    tainer (about 8 oz)
Part-skim ricotta—1 small con-
    tainer (about 15 oz)
Grated Parmesan—1 small bag
    or container (about 5 oz)
Eggs—3

Fruits

Blueberries—4 pints fresh (or 3
    12-oz bags frozen)
Bananas—2 medium (about 5
    inches)
Apples—2 medium

Lime—1
Lemon—1
Red or purple grapes—1 bunch
Oranges—2
Pink Florida grapefruits—2

Vegetables

Spinach—2 10-oz bags pre-washed
Broccoli—2 heads (about 3
    pounds total)
Baby carrots—1 16-oz bag
Mushrooms—1 10-oz package
Peppers—2, any color
Baking potatoes—2 medium
    (about 4 inches)

Green beans—4 oz (or 1 9-oz
    box frozen)
Zucchini—2 medium
Sweet potato—1 medium (about
    4 inches)
Onions—2 medium
Lettuce—1 small head (or 1 10-
    oz bag pre-washed)
Tomato—1 medium

Breads

Sesame breadsticks—2 individ-
    ual (look for breadsticks that
    are about 10 inches long and
    ½ inch in diameter)

Whole-grain bread—4 slices
Whole-wheat pitas—3

Meat and Fish

Skinless chicken breast—1 5-oz
    piece and 1 3-oz piece
Salmon—1 6-oz piece
Sirloin tips—1 4-oz piece
Shrimp—3 oz

Orange roughy—6-oz piece
    (orange roughy is a white fish
    from New Zealand—if you
    can't find it, substitute scrod
    or halibut)

Other

Hummus—1 7-oz container

Corn tortillas—1 small package of
6-inch tortillas (about 10 oz)

Miscellaneous

Ground flaxseed—can be found
at your local health food
store; buy the seeds whole
and grind them yourself or
buy preground flaxseed meal

Soy nuts—1 small package
(about 5 oz) (if you can't find
these at your local supermarket, try a health food store)

Soy bars—2, any flavor

Beverages

Green tea—one small box (about
20 teabags)

Herbal tea—one small box, any
flavor (about 20 tea bags)

Sparkling water—2 one-liter bottles (sparkling water is natural
spring water that is naturally
bubbly or with some added
mild carbonation)

Seltzer water—1 two-liter bottle
(seltzer is simply carbonated
water)

Low-calorie drinks—1 small bottle, your choice (try Snapple
diet lemonade or orange-
carrot drink, Crystal Light or
diet caffeine-free sodas)

Iced tea—1 small 3-oz jar instant
or 2 16-oz bottles ready-
made

Cranberry juice—1 small 6-oz
bottle or 1 8.45-oz juice box

Seasonings

Fajita seasoning—1 small
package

Ginger-teriyaki sauce—1 bottle
(I like the sauce by Rice
Road)

Italian seasoning—1 small
package (Good Seasons)

Cajun seasoning—1 small jar

Day 1

Breakfast

Anti-Aging Oatmeal
Green tea with a splash of orange juice

Anti-Aging Oatmeal
½ cup quick-cooking oatmeal
4 ounces skim milk
1 tablespoon ground flaxseed
Dash of cinnamon
½ cup fresh or frozen blueberries

Put oatmeal, milk, flaxseed and cinnamon in a microwave-safe bowl. Stir and cook as directed on the oatmeal canister. Top with the blueberries. This is my favorite way to start the day!

CALORIES	FAT	PROTEIN	FIBER	CALCIUM
214	5.3 g	9.2 g	6.7 g	194.1 mg

Midmorning Snack

Banana Split
8-ounce glass of sparkling water

Banana Split
1 8-ounce container of vanilla yogurt
1 5-inch banana

Slice banana and mix with yogurt.

CALORIES	FAT	PROTEIN	FIBER	CALCIUM
305	0.5 g	11.2 g	2.7 g	357 mg

Lunch

Spicy Soy Burger
Apple
8-ounce low-calorie beverage

Spicy Soy Burger
1 soy (or veggie) burger
2 slices whole-grain bread
½ cup spinach leaves
¼ cup salsa

Cook soy burger according to package directions. Place on one slice of whole-grain bread and top with spinach leaves, salsa and remaining slice of bread.

CALORIES	FAT	PROTEIN	FIBER	CALCIUM
312	2.75 g	25.5 g	8.2 g	88.5 mg

Midafternoon Snack

Nutty-Os
8-ounce glass of water with a splash of lime juice

Nutty-Os
1 cup Multi-Grain Cheerios
2 tablespoons almonds

Nibble on the Cheerios and almonds mixed together. This is a treat that isn't just for kids!

CALORIES	FAT	PROTEIN	FIBER	CALCIUM
276	15.35 g	8.6 g	5.35 g	180 mg

Dinner

Spring Chicken Stir-Fry
Green tea with lemon

Spring Chicken Stir-Fry
5 ounces skinless chicken breast, cut into ½-inch cubes
1 tablespoon olive oil
½ teaspoon minced garlic
½ teaspoon grated ginger
½ cup chopped broccoli
½ cup chopped carrots
½ cup chopped mushrooms
½ cup chopped peppers
1 cup cooked brown rice

Sauté the chicken in the olive oil with the garlic and ginger for 4 minutes. Add broccoli, carrots, mushrooms and peppers. Cook until vegetables are tender. Serve over the brown rice.

CALORIES	FAT	PROTEIN	FIBER	CALCIUM
639.5	20.84 g	46.1 g	7.32 g	79.05 mg

If you're following the **1,600-calorie plan,** make the following changes:

Dinner
Use 4 ounces of chicken
Use two-thirds cup of brown rice

TOTAL	1,800-CALORIE MEAL PLAN	1,600-CALORIE MEAL PLAN
CALORIES	1,826	1,639
FAT	44.3 grams (22%)	43.5 grams (24%)
PROTEIN	100.64 grams (22%)	88.54 grams (22%)
FIBER	30.2 grams	29.7 grams
CALCIUM	1,098.6 milligrams	888.2 milligrams

Day 2

Breakfast

Get-Up-and-Go Quickie
Green tea with a splash of cranberry juice

Get-Up-and-Go Quickie
1 slice whole-grain bread
1 tablespoon chunky peanut butter
1 cup red or purple grapes

Toast bread and top with peanut butter. Serve with grapes.

CALORIES	FAT	PROTEIN	FIBER	CALCIUM
214	9.3 g	7.45 g	3.95 g	34.5 mg

Midmorning Snack

Fruit "Take Five"
Herbal tea

Fruit "Take Five"
5 dried apricots
5 prunes
¼ cup golden raisins
Splash of Florida orange juice
Dash of cinnamon

Mix together apricots, prunes, raisins, orange juice and cinnamon and heat over low temperature until soft. Serve immediately.

CALORIES	FAT	PROTEIN	FIBER	CALCIUM
255	3 g	0.5 g	6 g	48.6 mg

Lunch

Vegetater
Orange
8-ounce glass sparkling water

Vegetater

1 5-ounce baked potato
½ cup broccoli
½ cup shredded light cheddar cheese

Top baked potato with broccoli and cheese. Place under broiler until cheese melts. Slice the orange and serve for dessert.

CALORIES	FAT	PROTEIN	FIBER	CALCIUM
459	10.9 g	31.1 g	10.8 g	624 mg

Midafternoon Snack

Mideast Afternoon
8-ounce glass seltzer

Mideast Afternoon

½ cup hummus
10 baby carrots

Enjoy this great Middle Eastern dip with carrots instead of chips. This snack always perks me up!

CALORIES	FAT	PROTEIN	FIBER	CALCIUM
241	10.5 g	6.7 g	8.45 g	80 mg

Dinner

Ragin' Cajun Salmon with Couscous
Iced tea with lemon

Ragin' Cajun Salmon with Couscous

1 6-ounce piece salmon filet
Cajun seasoning
1 cup couscous
1 cup green beans
1 teaspoon olive oil
½ teaspoon minced garlic

Coat the salmon in Cajun spices and broil, about 3 or 4 minutes on each side for a ½-inch thick piece (cooking time will vary depending on the thickness of the fish). Cook the couscous according to package directions. Sauté the green beans in the olive oil and garlic. Place the couscous on a plate and top with the fish, add the green beans and enjoy!

CALORIES	FAT	PROTEIN	FIBER	CALCIUM
652.5	24.8 g	46.35 g	6.5 g	86 mg

If you're following the **1,600-calorie plan,** make the following changes:

Lunch
Use a 4-ounce potato

Dinner
Use 4 ounces of salmon

TOTAL	1,800-CALORIE MEAL PLAN	1,600-CALORIE MEAL PLAN
CALORIES	1,821	1,660
FAT	61.2 grams (30%)	55 grams (30%)
PROTEIN	91.5 grams (21%)	84.5 grams (20%)
FIBER	35.7 grams	35.1 grams
CALCIUM	871 milligrams	869 milligrams

Breakfast

Sunrise Smoothie

Sunrise Smoothie
8 ounces skim milk
1 8-ounce container lemon yogurt
½ cup blueberries
1 tablespoon ground flaxseed

Blend all of the ingredients until smooth. Pour, drink and dive into a great day.

CALORIES	FAT	PROTEIN	FIBER	CALCIUM
356	3.3 g	19.6 g	4.25 g	689.5 mg

Midmorning Snack

Toast Tops
8-ounce glass seltzer

Toast Tops
1 slice whole-grain bread
1 tablespoon chunky peanut butter

Toast bread and top with peanut butter—a great energy booster!

CALORIES	FAT	PROTEIN	FIBER	CALCIUM
180	9.7 g	5.95 g	2.15 g	18.5 mg

Lunch

Pizza Pizzazz
Iced tea with lime

Pizza Pizzazz

1 whole-wheat pita
¼ cup chunky pizza sauce
½ cup raw spinach leaves
½ cup shredded part-skim mozzarella

Divide pita into two halves. Top each half with equal amounts of pizza sauce, spinach leaves and cheese. Broil until cheese melts.

CALORIES	FAT	PROTEIN	FIBER	CALCIUM
350	13.9 g	15.5 g	6.1 g	301.5 mg

Midafternoon Snack

Nutri-Nibbles
Ice water

Nutri-Nibbles

½ cup roasted soy nuts
½ cup golden raisins

Snack on these nutrient-packed nuts and raisins for instant energy.

CALORIES	FAT	PROTEIN	FIBER	CALCIUM
351	6.3 g	19.9 g	9.7 g	119.4 mg

Dinner

Fajita Fun
Florida orange Juice with Seltzer

Fajita Fun

1 4-ounce piece sirloin tip, thinly sliced
2 teaspoons olive oil
Fajita seasonings
½ cup thinly sliced red and green peppers
½ cup thinly sliced onion
2 corn tortillas
2 tablespoons salsa

Sauté sirloin and fajita seasonings in olive oil. When the meat is done, remove it from the heat and in the same pan sauté peppers and onions until slightly soft. Add meat back to the pan and heat for 1 minute. Divide equally between two corn tortillas. Add 1 tablespoon salsa to each tortilla. Roll up and eat.

Orange Juice with Seltzer

3 ounces calcium-fortified Florida orange juice
3 ounces seltzer

Mix seltzer and orange juice for a refreshing drink.

CALORIES	FAT	PROTEIN	FIBER	CALCIUM
566	17.3 g	38.6 g	6.2 g	342 mg

If you're following the **1,600-calorie plan**, make the following changes:

Midafternoon Snack

Have ¼ cup each soy nuts and raisins

Dinner

Drink plain seltzer—skip the orange juice

TOTAL	1,800-CALORIE MEAL PLAN	1,600-CALORIE MEAL PLAN
CALORIES	1,803	1,596
FAT	47.5 grams (24%)	41.3 grams (23%)
PROTEIN	99.6 grams (22%)	92.9 grams (23%)
FIBER	28.4 grams	25.2 grams
CALCIUM	1,431.1 milligrams	1,231 milligrams

Day 4

Breakfast

Oatmeal Berry Cobbler

Oatmeal Berry Cobbler
½ cup uncooked oatmeal
1 tablespoon brown sugar
Dash cinnamon
1 teaspoon whipped butter
1 cup blueberries
¼ cup Craisins
Splash of orange juice
1 8-ounce container vanilla yogurt

Mix together oatmeal, brown sugar, cinnamon and butter until crumbs form. In a baking pan mix together blueberries, Craisins and orange juice. Top with the crumb mixture and bake at 350 degrees for 15 minutes. Top with vanilla yogurt.

CALORIES	FAT	PROTEIN	FIBER	CALCIUM
610	7.8 g	15.5 g	8.7 g	378 mg

Midmorning Snack

1 soy bar
1 cup tea

CALORIES	FAT	PROTEIN	FIBER	CALCIUM
230	5 g	14 g	2 g	250 mg

Lunch

Tuna Wrap
Orange
8-ounce glass sparkling water

Tuna Wrap
1 3-ounce can water-packed tuna
1 tablespoon light mayonnaise
¼ cup shredded lettuce
1 whole-wheat pita

Mix together tuna and light mayonnaise. Stuff tuna and lettuce into pita bread.

CALORIES	FAT	PROTEIN	FIBER	CALCIUM
394	9.4 g	28.1 g	8.3 g	93 mg

Midafternoon Snack

Carrots 'n' Dip
8-ounce glass water with lemon

Carrots 'n' Dip
½ cup fat-free bean dip
10 baby carrots

A midday twist on chips and dip.

CALORIES	FAT	PROTEIN	FIBER	CALCIUM
141	0.3 g	8 g	8.4 g	62 mg

Dinner

Rainbow Kabobs
Sweet Potato Wedges
Green tea

Rainbow Kabobs
1 3-ounce piece skinless chicken, cut into cubes
1 cup mixed zucchini, mushrooms and yellow peppers, cut into chunks
Low-calorie ginger teriyaki sauce

Thread chicken and veggies on a skewer and allow to marinate in the ginger teriyaki sauce for at least 1 hour. Heat up the grill and cook the kabob until the chicken is cooked through, about 7 minutes per side, depending on the thickness of the chicken.

Sweet Potato Wedges
1 sweet potato, cut into wedges
1 tablespoon olive oil

Brush the sweet potato wedges with olive oil and bake at 450 degrees until done, about 40 to 45 minutes.

CALORIES	FAT	PROTEIN	FIBER	CALCIUM
486	19.6 g	39.6 g	6.8 g	66 mg

If you're following the **1,600-calorie plan**, make the following changes:

Breakfast
Have 4 ounces of yogurt; skip the Craisins

Dinner
Use 2 teaspoons olive oil instead of 1 tablespoon

TOTAL	1,800-CALORIE MEAL PLAN	1,600-CALORIE MEAL PLAN
CALORIES	1,861	1,622
FAT	42.1 grams (20%)	37.7 grams (21%)
PROTEIN	105.2 grams (23%)	100.2 grams (25%)
FIBER	34.2 grams	33.2 grams
CALCIUM	849 milligrams	674 milligrams

Breakfast

Sunrise Sandwich
½ pink Florida grapefruit
Seltzer water with a splash of orange juice

Sunrise Sandwich

1 soy patty
1 slice light cheddar cheese
1 tablespoon salsa
1 mini whole-wheat pita

Cook the soy patty according to package directions. Top with cheddar cheese. Slide into pita and add salsa. A spicy start to a new day!

CALORIES	FAT	PROTEIN	FIBER	CALCIUM
388	6.8 g	32.5 g	9.6 g	279.5 mg

Midmorning Snack

2 low-fat cinnamon or honey-oat granola bars
1 cup green tea

CALORIES	FAT	PROTEIN	FIBER	CALCIUM
200	6 g	4 g	3 g	0 mg

Lunch

Seafood Spinach Salad
2 sesame breadsticks
Seltzer water

Seafood Spinach Salad

2 cups baby spinach leaves
1 3-ounce can salmon
½ cup mandarin oranges
2 tablespoons chopped walnuts
2 tablespoons citrus vinaigrette

Toss together spinach, salmon, mandarin oranges, and walnuts. Dress with citrus vinaigrette. Serve with breadsticks.

CALORIES	FAT	PROTEIN	FIBER	CALCIUM
446	26.1 g	25.4 g	4.6 g	329 mg

Midafternoon Snack

Berries à la Mode
Ice water

Berries à la Mode
½ cup berries
1 8-ounce container vanilla yogurt

Place berries in a bowl and top with yogurt.

CALORIES	FAT	PROTEIN	FIBER	CALCIUM
240	0 g	10 g	2 g	354.5 mg

Dinner

Shrimp Shape-up
Green tea

Shrimp Shape-up
1½ cups pasta
3 ounces shrimp
1 tablespoon olive oil
½ teaspoon minced garlic
1 cup steamed broccoli

Cook pasta according to package directions and set aside. Sauté shrimp in olive oil with minced garlic until pink. Add shrimp and steamed broccoli to the pasta. Serve piping hot!

CALORIES	FAT	PROTEIN	FIBER	CALCIUM
556	16.4 g	33.6 g	9.2 g	142 mg

If you're following the **1,600-calorie plan**, make the following changes:

Midmorning
Eat 1 granola bar instead of 2

Dinner
Use 1 teaspoon olive oil

TOTAL	1,800-CALORIE MEAL PLAN	1,600-CALORIE MEAL PLAN
CALORIES	1,830	1,647
FAT	55.3 grams (27%)	43.5 grams (23%)
PROTEIN	105.5 grams (23%)	103.5 grams (25%)
FIBER	28.4 grams	26.9 grams
CALCIUM	1,105 milligrams	1,105 milligrams

Day 6

Breakfast

Super Cereal
Green tea with lemon

Super Cereal

1 cup Multi-Grain Cheerios
1 tablespoon ground flaxseed
1 5-inch banana, sliced
8 ounces skim milk

Place Cheerios in a bowl. Top with flaxseed and banana. Pour in the milk and start eating.

CALORIES	FAT	PROTEIN	FIBER	CALCIUM
331	4.8 g	12.6 g	7.9 g	442 mg

Midmorning Snack

1 soy bar
1 cup green tea

CALORIES	FAT	PROTEIN	FIBER	CALCIUM
230	5 g	14 g	2 g	250 mg

Lunch

Popeye's Pasta
Apple
8-ounce glass sparkling water

Popeye's Pasta

½ cup frozen spinach, thawed
½ cup part-skim ricotta
2 jumbo pasta shells (cooked)
½ cup chunky tomato sauce
2 tablespoons grated Parmesan cheese

Mix together spinach and ricotta. Divide equally and spoon into pasta shells. Add sauce and cheese. Place in a baking dish, cover with foil and bake at 350 degrees for 15 minutes.

CALORIES	FAT	PROTEIN	FIBER	CALCIUM
518	15.1 g	34.2 g	9.4 g	664.7 mg

Midafternoon Snack

Very Berry Smoothie

Very Berry Smoothie

½ cup berries (your choice)
4 ounces skim milk
6 ounces calcium-fortified orange juice

Blend together all three ingredients until smooth. Pour and enjoy!

CALORIES	FAT	PROTEIN	FIBER	CALCIUM
170	0 g	4 g	2 g	362.5 mg

Dinner

Frittata Italiano
Potato Wedges
Iced tea with lime

Frittata Italiano

¼ cup zucchini, chopped
¼ cup mushrooms, chopped
¼ cup peppers, chopped
1 teaspoon olive oil
½ teaspoon minced garlic
3 eggs
2 tablespoons water
Dash of pepper
Dash Italian seasoning
1 tablespoon grated Parmesan cheese

Sauté zucchini, mushrooms and peppers in olive oil and garlic. In a separate bowl beat eggs with water. Pour egg mixture over vegetables. Sprinkle with pepper, Italian seasoning and cheese. Cook on low heat until set.

Potato Wedges

1 4-ounce baked potato
2 teaspoons olive oil

Cut potato into wedges and sauté with olive oil in a small pan until hot.

CALORIES	FAT	PROTEIN	FIBER	CALCIUM
516	26.2 g	24.9 g	3.5 g	161.5 mg

If you're following the **1,600-calorie plan**, make the following changes:

Breakfast
Skip the flaxseed

Lunch
Skip the apple

Dinner
Use 2 teaspoons olive oil instead of 3

TOTAL	1,800-CALORIE MEAL PLAN	1,600-CALORIE MEAL PLAN
CALORIES	1,830	1,603
FAT	51.1 grams (25%)	45.9 grams (26%)
PROTEIN	89.7 grams (23%)	89.3 grams (22%)
FIBER	24.9 grams	21.2 grams
CALCIUM	1,880.7 milligrams	1,870.7 milligrams

Breakfast

Weightless Waffles
8-ounce glass skim milk

Weightless Waffles

½ cup blueberries
2 whole-grain waffles
¼ cup light syrup

Toast waffles and top with blueberries and syrup.

CALORIES	FAT	PROTEIN	FIBER	CALCIUM
408	6 g	13 g	6 g	360.5 mg

Midmorning Snack

1 pink grapefruit
1 cup green tea

CALORIES	FAT	PROTEIN	FIBER	CALCIUM
80	0.2 g	1.6 g	2.8 g	30 mg

Lunch

Power Pasta
8-ounce glass seltzer water

Power Pasta

1 cup dry wheat pasta
½ cup broccoli
½ cup part-skim ricotta
2 tablespoons grated Parmesan cheese
1 small tomato, sliced

Cook pasta according to package directions. While pasta is cooking, steam broccoli. Drain pasta and add broccoli, ricotta and Parmesan. Toss until thoroughly mixed. Serve with sliced tomato.

CALORIES	FAT	PROTEIN	FIBER	CALCIUM
483	14.7 g	30.6 g	8.3 g	565 mg

Midafternoon Snack

Stay-Young Snack
Iced green tea

Stay-Young Snack
½ cup roasted soy nuts
⅓ cup Craisins

CALORIES	FAT	PROTEIN	FIBER	CALCIUM
250	4 g	12 g	7 g	60 mg

Dinner

Down-Under Dinner
Herbal tea

Down-Under Dinner
1 6-ounce piece orange roughy
½ cup thinly sliced onions
1 cup spicy stewed tomatoes
2 cups fresh spinach leaves
2 teaspoons olive oil
Dash black pepper
½ teaspoon minced garlic
1 cup cooked brown rice

Place fish in ovenproof dish. Top with onions and tomatoes. Cover with foil and bake at 350 degrees for 20 minutes or until fish flakes. While fish is cooking, sauté spinach with olive oil, pepper and garlic. Serve with brown rice.

CALORIES	FAT	PROTEIN	FIBER	CALCIUM
604	15.3 g	43.1 g	10.1 g	292 mg

If you're following the **1,600-calorie plan**, make the following changes:

Breakfast
Have 1 waffle and 2 tablespoons of syrup

Lunch
Use 1 tablespoon Parmesan cheese

Midafternoon Snack

Have ¼ cup Craisins

TOTAL	1,800-CALORIE MEAL PLAN	1,600-CALORIE MEAL PLAN
CALORIES	1,825	1,628
FAT	41.6 grams (20%)	37.1 grams (20%)
PROTEIN	98.9 grams (22%)	94.3 grams (23%)
FIBER	34.2 grams	32.2 grams
CALCIUM	1,307.5 milligrams	1,217.5 milligrams

5

Health: Body Sense for Women

Standard Size

I bought myself a bikini
to celebrate
my 46th summer.

Like a diamond
flashing its flaws
at the hot sun
I stood out,
no longer the standard
18th summer size.

At least
there is no standard size for spirit,
and how lovely mine has grown.
My spirit
unlike my body
has no visible shape.
It can not be judged
by the ordinary eye.
I bought myself a bikini
to celebrate
my 46th summer.
I am showing off my spirit.

—MARILYN BECKER

This lovely poem is a wonderful expression of healthy self-satisfaction, a celebration of the writer's mental and physical well-being. I happily share her delight in our post-40 selves. I was surprised to discover that this birthday was much less of a wrenching life experience than turning 30. At 40 many things in your life have settled into place. You feel more confident, more comfortable about yourself. But it's also important to feel good *inside* yourself—strong and healthy. I know I do, and I plan to continue feeling that way. . . . Think positive!

Still, I recognize that the person I am today may need a little more attention than my younger self. Although I have always exercised regularly and paid attention to what I eat, now that I've passed that "big" birthday I can't take my health as much for granted as I could as a teenager (or even a 28- or 38-year-old). As you age, good health is less a matter of luck and more a matter of making smart choices. You have to take preventive measures and be more disciplined about health-related issues. The payoff is enormous. Happily, at 40 you are still young enough to establish patterns that will help give you many years of health and happiness. Plan to age like a gorgeous classic car: You may require a little more maintenance as the years go by, but you can look good enough to turn heads and you can still keep rolling along.

Seize the moment. Take a breath, get that oxygen flowing and resolve to start today. You can do it!

We've already talked about weight and diet. You know how important these two factors are to your appearance, but they also have a lot to do with your health. For every inch your waistline exceeds the size of your chest, you can deduct two years from your life expectancy. Of course, many diseases are related to excess weight—stroke and heart disease, along with certain kinds of cancer, are only a few. And if you thought beauty sleep was a luxury, think again. New research shows that lack of quality sleep can actually result in premature aging.

Eating too much, burning the candle at both ends—we all have our vices. As a teenager living near the beach, I baked myself like a rotisserie chicken, and I still love that ol' sun. But preparing for a healthy old age means cutting down on—or cutting out—what's bad for us, whether it's bacon double cheeseburgers, substituting caffeine for sleep, or acquiring a deep tan.

We also have to do more of what's good for us: more fish and vegetables, more rest, more sunblock and hats with brims. Plus there are new things to think about. Prime example: those monthly breast self-exams. I have to admit that I'm not absolutely religious about making them happen. (Blame a mixture of apprehension and a hectic lifestyle.) But we all should be working on substituting new and better habits for our old, bad ones.

Health: Body Sense for Women

We would like to think that lung cancer, breast tumors and diabetes are heath problems that happen to other people. But of course, that's not so. If you're lucky, you'll get some warning that there's a problem: Perhaps you'll start to feel fatigued and discover your thyroid needs a boost, or you'll discover a tiny lump in your breast that turns out to be benign. But if you don't make a point of watching your health, and if you don't happen to get that wake-up call, you may not discover that something is wrong until you're at the point where nothing can be done. You don't want that to happen. So it's extremely important that you do what you can to avoid health problems.

Be proactive. Take steps now to head off health problems before they start. Very small changes can turn out to be lifesavers. You've got years ahead to see those changes pay off, and it's critical you make time for them—starting right now.

Women are programmed to be caregivers. We all have tons of responsibilities—to our kids, husband, parents, relatives, business associates, friends and neighbors. We all find time to do the caretaking, to do our jobs, to volunteer at the school or the community association, to keep the house in order and to decorate for the holidays. What's last on the list? Too often it's you. I know lots of women who treat their pets better than they treat themselves. Most of us wouldn't dream of feeding Fido a steady diet of junk food and cigarettes or neglect to take the dog for walks. We wouldn't fail to schedule Fluffy's annual checkup. So why are we so neglectful of our own well-being? The easy answer is that we simply don't have the time.

Well, you've heard it before, and I'll say it again: You have only one body, and you have to take care of it. If you want to be there for your loved ones, if you want to dance at your child's wedding and play with your grandchildren and go on that cruise you've always dreamed of— even if you just want to be around to see to it that Fido and Fluffy are well taken care of—you have to invest some time and energy into caring for yourself. You won't be able to nurture anyone if you don't nurture yourself. You can't contribute to your family's well-being if you yourself are ill. Time spent on taking care of yourself isn't time taken away from others; rather, it's time dedicated to ensuring that you'll be there for those who love and depend on you. By caring for yourself, you're caring for them. You can't argue with that!

According to the National Institute on Aging, about one-fifth of people over age 65 have physical limitations that prevent them from accomplishing everyday activities such as driving, bathing or even getting dressed. I don't want you to be one of them! To avoid spending your retirement years confined to a wheelchair or as a resident of a nursing home, it's important to learn as much as you can about your health and to take a few basic precautions.

While your genes may put you at higher risk for illnesses such as heart disease and cancer, family history is not the whole story even in those cases. There is no reason to be a fatalist about your prospects for good health. Experts say that the *majority* of serious health problems are caused by not taking proper care of your body. As my good friend and physical fitness pioneer Jack LaLanne says, "People don't die of old age—they die of neglect."

I've already discussed the power of exercise and eating right. But there's more to staying healthy than weight training and vitamins. You need to incorporate some other routines into your life. You have to have body sense.

SIX BODY-SENSE STRATEGIES

If you say you're confused by all the conflicting health information in the news, I wouldn't be surprised. In fact, if you are *not* confused, you're probably not paying enough attention. Every time you turn on the TV or read a magazine, there seems to be a report on a new study that contradicts the findings of previous one. I have training in the health field, and even I have trouble keeping it all straight!

While the media do a good job of keeping us informed about new studies, they don't always put information in perspective. Every individual study has to be interpreted in light of all the other information that currently exists in the particular area. To help set things straight for you, I've talked to experts from the American Heart Association, the American Cancer Society and other top authorities. I've asked them what works and what doesn't, what's harmful and what's helpful, and I've used their answers to develop six simple strategies for defending yourself against long-range health problems.

If you're the kind of person who gives thought to her health—and you must be or you wouldn't be reading this book—you will probably discover that some of the anti-aging essentials discussed on the following pages are already part of your life. If so, it won't be much trouble to add a few more. If not, make a resolution to start. They're crucial to keeping you at the top of your form.

1. Reduce Stress

According to the people who tabulate such things, the average person in business deals with 32 phone calls, 14 E-mails , 11 voice mails and 9 faxes each day! Just juggling all that input is a lot of pressure. And you may be dealing with high-pressure situations many other times in the day. I know what it's like to have a crazy morning getting the kids off to school, or dealing with a sick relative's caretaker, and then having the computer screen freeze up in the middle of a big job. The accumulated effect of many such incidents can have a tremendous effect on your physical health. According to the American Institute of Stress, 75 to 90 percent of all visits to primary-care physicians are stress-related complaints.

The stress response—sometimes called the "fight-or-flight" response—enables humans to deal with brief physical changes. Your body releases hormones such as adrenaline and cortisol to increase your blood pressure and give you extra energy. This set of physiological responses was Mother Nature's way of giving an instant shot of get-up-and-go to our ancestors in an emergency situation like a face-to-face encounter with a man-eating tiger.

You probably won't run into any tigers today, but you may have to deal with a copy machine that eats your documents, a washing machine that eats your socks and a transmission problem that eats your auto budget. In response, your heart thumps. Your muscles tense. Your blood vessels constrict. Your hands tremble. Your face gets hot. You start to perspire. In the stressful world we live in, our bodies may activate the stress response chronically and often in response to psychological stressors. This can cause a variety of short- and long-term problems.

Minor and common side effects of stress include pounding headaches, irritability, insomnia or tiredness. A recent poll by *Redbook* magazine reported that stress is the number-one reason women feel fatigued. It has been linked to hair loss and gum disease. Stress can cause you to grind your teeth at night, set off a case of hives or eczema or send you to the refrigerator on a regular basis.

Worse, constant stress can result in serious, long-term consequences. Because it weakens your immune system, stress can make you more vulnerable to colds and can cause wounds to heal more slowly. Scientists have found that stress-related diseases include depression, hypertension, atherosclerosis, ulcers, colitis and reproductive dysfunction. One recent study links emotional stress caused by the loss of a loved one to an increased risk of early death from heart disease or cancer. Another suggests that people who suffer workplace stress are more likely to have a disorder in the body's clot-dissolving system that can lead to the buildup of fatty deposits in the arteries.

Even if such devastating long-term effects don't shorten your life, stress can reduce its quality. When you are constantly stressed, you can't enjoy your life. But I can guess what you're thinking when you read that you should reduce stress. "Impossible," you say to yourself. "I'm dealing with [choose one or more] teenage children, a difficult boss, a parent with Alzheimer's" and on and on. We all have big, real-life problems.

Maybe we can't take away the problem, but we can learn some coping techniques to reduce the impact of stress on your body. These are some of my favorite strategies:

Back off. When you start feeling stressed in any particular situation, stop, if you can, and ask yourself: "Is this situation truly important? Can I distance myself from it? Can I get control of it in any way? Is there good reason to spend energy getting upset about it?" If you have many or chronic stressful situations to deal with, would it be helpful for you to learn meditation techniques? Or could you get some counseling?

Get moving. A recent report in the *Annals of Behavioral Medicine* confirms what dedicated exercisers like me have known for years: Working out can help reduce the physical effects of daily stress. Whether the exercise is a peppy jog or a soothing yoga routine, it will release mood-boosting hormones called endorphins that help chase away your worries. Whenever I can feel myself getting anxious—the airline lost my bag, the heating system has gone on the fritz again, or I'm going to have to argue with the customer service rep at the utility company—I try to force myself to take a break. I do some neck exercises, or I stand and do some stretches. Better yet, if possible I head outside and take a quick walk. Physical movement takes my mind off my problems and also gives my muscles a workout. That's the beauty of exercise—it's good for you in so many ways!

Slow down. Meditate. The simple act of sitting quietly and clearing your mind of to-do lists, bills to pay, deadlines and all other thoughts has been shown to reduce the physical effects of stress and anxiety. For stress maintenance, try to meditate for at least five minutes daily. Find a peaceful place and use deep, controlled breathing to draw your consciousness inward and away from your everyday cares. Focus on a single object, such as a burning candle, or repeat a phrase in your head to keep your mind from wandering. This isn't the time to start planning your Thanksgiving menu or have an imaginary conversation with the friend who hurt your feelings. It's a time to let all of that negative energy go. I like meditating at the end of a tough day, right before bedtime. Before I know it, my body is relaxed, and I'm sinking into a blissful slumber.

Breathe deeply. If you haven't time for a full-fledged meditation, try this shortcut for any occasion when you feel anxious—before you have to make a presentation to your boss, say, or while you're waiting to see the doctor. To slow down your racing heart and relax your body, take a few deep, long breaths. Draw the air into your abdomen, not the upper part of your chest. Feel your belly expand as you inhale, then release all that pent-up stress as you exhale. Within a minute you should feel the tension lessening. At the end of the chapter I describe breathing exercises for different kinds of stressful situations.

Write it down. Many studies have shown that putting your problems and concerns down on paper can help reduce stress and improve your outlook on life. Spend 5 to 10 minutes each day writing your deepest thoughts and emotions in a journal. Many people find it useful to write a quick letter to yourself outlining your feelings when there is an immediate crisis such as a fight with your sister or being told by your boss that there will be no raises this year. Writing down your thoughts helps you think more clearly and also gets the negative emotions out of your system.

Do a good deed. Turn negatives into positives by doing something kind for someone else. It can be something as small as helping an elderly person cross the street or assisting someone in the supermarket. I always help moms with strollers—I've been there. Go through your address book and call a friend you haven't heard from in a while, just to say hello. Write a little "I love you" on a piece of paper and put it in your husband's briefcase or suitcase for his next trip. It's a nice surprise. Copy an old photograph and send it to family members. The best gifts cost little and, what's more, give you something back by raising your spirits.

Laugh out loud. Patch Adams isn't the only one who believes in the healing power of laughter. Studies have found that humor can help reduce tension and improve immune function. Some doctors have recommended that patients turn to humor as a relief for everything from depression to cancer. *I Love Lucy* reruns always get me giggling, or I rent a favorite comedy. Any essay from any Dave Barry book is usually good for a laugh.

Talk it out. I've been blessed with a mother, three sisters, a brother and a husband who have been good listeners. I also have good friends with whom I share my life. When I'm feeling overwhelmed by work or have had some bad news, I turn to them for emotional support. Just knowing that they are there makes me feel better instantly. And in turn, I always want to be there for them. Talking out your problems helps you come up with rational solutions instead of just feeling overwhelmed. If you're having a major crisis such as a divorce or serious illness, consider finding a counselor who can listen and give advice. Another point of view, whether it comes from a friend or a professional, is immensely valuable.

2. Get More Sleep

In Gallup surveys, 56 percent of the adult population reports that drowsiness in the daytime is a problem. Do you constantly feel drained? Your body is trying to tell you something. Fatigue is a cry for help! We've all experienced the short-term effects of not getting enough shut-eye. It makes us tired, lethargic, cranky and unable to concentrate. We're more likely to have an accident or fall asleep at the wheel. Our skin looks dull and we develop big, dark circles under the eyes. But sleep doesn't simply improve our personality and make us look better.

Sleep is not a luxury and it is not a waste of time. It is an essential ingredient of a healthy, fit lifestyle. While you sleep, your body gets rid of waste products and circulates minerals, vitamins and hormones. During sleep your body produces most of the infection-fighting substances that help you recover from illness and injury. It also produces the natural human growth hormone that maintains and repairs muscles. If we don't maintain our muscles, our metabolism slows down (and we all know what happens then!)

Cutting back on sleep has many consequences. Lack of sleep increases the incidence of all kinds of illnesses, from the common cold to more serious immune-deficiency disorders, and it may hasten the onset of ailments such as hypertension and memory loss. It upsets the body's metabolism in the same fashion as aging. A new study from the University of Chicago shows that sleep-deprived bodies are less efficient at metabolizing sugar, leading to elevated glucose levels that are linked to dangerous conditions such as diabetes, high blood pressure and obesity.

All this is meant to make you aware that getting enough sleep is critical to enjoying good health. Even if you're religious about exercising and following a sensible diet, you won't get the full benefits of all your hard work if you don't get your ZZZs. Cut out something else—that late-night movie, perhaps?—but don't skimp on the shut-eye. If you haven't been getting enough, you'll notice the difference right away. You'll feel better, look better and be able to engage in life with renewed energy.

Of course, not all sleep is good sleep, and experts say quality is just as important as quantity. A night of fitful tossing and turning doesn't give you the same benefits as eight hours of restful snoozing. So take the time to create a sleep-friendly environment. Here are seven strategies for achieving a good night's rest:

Skip the caffeine. Avoid caffeine and other stimulants for at least six hours before your scheduled bedtime. This means no coffee, no cola, no tea and no chocolate. And check medicine labels. Some over-the-counter headache medications are loaded with caffeine.

Try some warm milk. This time-honored remedy has a scientific basis. Milk is rich in tryptophan, an amino acid that may help you go to sleep.

Take a warm shower or bath. Warm water can help you relax by relieving tension and soothing tired muscles, which creates a calming effect. Don't do this right before you crawl under the covers, however. Take a half-hour bath a couple of hours before you plan to retire. The cooldown leads to drowsiness.

Don't hit the sack until you're ready to sleep. Do not balance your checkbook in bed. Don't correct your management presentation in bed. Some people get drowsy watching TV or reading a book, but for obvious reasons avoid programs or books that are exciting or disturbing. Some experts even advise against TV and say your bed should be reserved for only one activity: sleeping. (Okay, TWO activities!) The idea is to get relaxed.

Stick to a routine. Our bodies respond to patterns. Try to go to bed at the same time each night and arise at the same time each morning. Sleeping late on weekends (or any day) disrupts sleep patterns and may leave you staring at the ceiling come nighttime. If you nap in the daytime, keep the nap to thirty minutes tops. After that point it turns into deep sleep.

Avoid alcohol. While a cocktail or two may help you fall asleep, you're apt to wake up several hours later, then toss and turn for the remainder of the night. Why? Alcohol alters your normal sleep patterns—not to mention those extra trips to the bathroom. No matter if you've spent eight hours in bed, you'll still feel tired and groggy the following day.

Keep it cool. A cool room is the best for sleeping, especially since our bodies become naturally drowsy as the temperature decreases. Open a window to let in some cool air or turn down the thermostat and the sandman will come in, too.

Try aromatherapy. Essential oils, lotions or an aromatherapy diffuser are wonderful sources of soothing scents. Researchers have found that lavender is especially effective for insomnia. Try a lavender eye pillow or eye mask.

If you have chronic sleep problems, don't shrug them off. Talk to your doctor. This may be caused by menopause, depression or other problems for which medical help may be available.

3. Stop Smoking

I'm lucky to have grown up in a family of nonsmokers. Yes, I lit up a cigarette in college (got dizzy and hated it). I feel sorry for the people who get hooked. The price you pay for smoking is enormous. Those little white sticks contain thousands of chemicals, including many that dramatically increase your risk for a host of life-threatening diseases. Among them are nicotine, a stimulant that not only keeps you addicted but also increases your blood pressure, and traces of poisons such as arsenic.

Smoking may lower blood levels of antioxidants, which (as I've explained in Chapter 4) protect against many of the diseases of aging. A Harvard Medical School study shows that women who smoke 35 or more cigarettes a day increase their risk of cataracts by 63 percent. If you smoke, your chance of developing lung cancer is 10 times greater than that of nonsmokers. You're two to six times more likely to suffer a heart attack. You're also at much greater risk of having a stroke or developing chronic bronchitis, emphysema or osteoporosis.

Most smokers know about the risk of fatal disease but figure it won't happen to them, or if it does, it will be years from now; so yes, they'll quit—someday. Many women claim to smoke to keep their weight down so they'll look more attractive. Do they think yellow teeth and stained fingers are pretty? Do they think wrinkles look good? Because smoking decreases blood flow to the skin, researchers calculate that it is second only to sunbathing as a cause of premature aging of the skin. Not to mention that when you smoke, your breath smells and your clothes stink. Believe me, people notice. Worst of all, you may be harming your loved ones. Up to 8,000 lung cancer deaths are attributed to secondhand smoke each year.

I know, I know. If you're smoking, the last thing you need is a lecture from me. You're tired of people telling you how bad smoking is and why you should stop. The best way to shut us up? Get help so you can rid yourself of this bad habit for good.

Even if you've been a chain-smoker for half your life, experts say that you can undo some of the damage done to your arteries and lungs by quitting now. Within one to three years of grinding out your last butt, your heart disease risk could be cut in half, and your risk for lung cancer and emphysema could be significantly lower. But that doesn't mean you can afford to wait a few years before stopping. Every time you light up, you make things a little bit worse.

Quitting is tough, but take heart: Many people have managed to do it. Whether you go cold turkey or slowly wean yourself off the cigarettes, you can help the process by chewing gum, drinking lots of water and taking deep breaths of fresh air. Many people also have success with nicotine patches, nicotine gum or alternative methods such as hypnosis. Talk to your doctor or consult the American Lung Association's "Quit Smoking Action Plan"(www.lungusa.org) to determine the best route for you.

And let me take away your one big excuse: that if you stop smoking, you'll gain a lot of weight. According to the Centers for Disease Control and Prevention in Atlanta, the average woman who quits gains no more than five pounds, and even that can be prevented through sensible eating and regular exercise.

4. Stay Out of the Sun

Direct sun exposure significantly increases your risk of skin cancer and cataracts. And if you want to know how well your skin will age, take into account your genes and how much time you spend catching the rays.

As I've already confessed, I was a sun junkie. I grew up on the California coast, and like the rest of my friends, I used to slather myself in oil and bask in the sunshine. I wouldn't dream of doing this today, but on the other hand, for active women like me, staying out of the sun entirely is virtually impossible.

It's also not a great idea. Everyone needs a little sun in her life. It lifts your spirits and it gives you a healthy dose of vitamin D. You can get your share on the golf course, walking around town or driving in the car with the top down. I believe in 15 to 20 minutes of outdoor sun without sunscreen and with some of your body parts, such as arms or legs, unclothed to soak in the good vitamin D. To be on the safe side, wear a wide-brimmed hat and sunglasses and long sleeves and pants when possible.

Cover all exposed areas—especially your face and neck—with sunscreen that has an SPF of at least 15. And before you apply that sunscreen, check the bottom of the bottle or tube for an expiration date (most brands have it now). There's no point applying sunscreen that lost its effectiveness in 1999.

Wearing a hat—and sunglasses, of course—also cuts your risk of cataracts, which are caused by frequent exposure to the sun's ultraviolet rays. In addition, scientists believe that vitamins C and E and carotenoids (most often found in dark green leafy vegetables) helps prevent cataracts, and all these are part of a healthy diet—another reason to eat right.

5. Get the Best Medical Care

You suddenly notice a little flap of skin under your arm and watch it nervously for months. Or you suffer weeks of feeling a little short of breath and worrying about it at night. Most likely your problem is a harmless skin tag caused by friction and the breathlessness is just the result of stress from your job, but why add a layer of extra worry? Worse yet, why take the risk that you've got a more serious problem that's being neglected? Go to a health care professional and get yourself checked out.

Having a regular checkup once a year is the best anxiety reliever I can think of. Instead of focusing solely on a single symptom, you can discuss all aspects of your health. In talking with you, your doctor can pick up on any changes in your health and lifestyle habits that you may not have noticed and order whatever tests are appropriate at your age. Having a regular consultation with a professional will help you take better care of yourself. If something unusual does subsequently turn up, you have the assurance that you've been checked recently and chances are you're okay; also, you'll have someone to turn to who's familiar with your medical history.

Give yourself a regular checkup as your birthday present to yourself. It'll make you feel great—and you'll never forget when you're next due.

Here are some ways to get the best medical care you can.

Choose the right doctor. If you feel comfortable with your doctor, you'll be more likely to go on a regular basis. Finding the right doctor may require some time and effort, but the results will be worth it. Get a referral from another doctor you trust and respect. If you're new to an area, call the local hospital and get a referral from the chief resident or the patient services department. Or check with trusted friends. When I moved to Washington, D.C., 17 years ago, Jeff and I were planning to start a family. I needed a good gynecologist and I wanted to make sure that I found the right person to deliver my babies. I didn't know anyone in the area, and I didn't just want to pick a name out of a directory. Finally, after I got to know a few women in my neighborhood, I got the names of two doctors who both sounded great.

But a recommendation from friends requires some extra checking. Most physicians who are affiliated with hospitals have been thoroughly checked out by the hospital board.

To investigate further, check with your state's medical certification board or try a Web site such as the American Medical Association's Doctor Finder (http://www.ama-assn.org/aps/amahg.htm).

Call the physician's office directly and ask some general questions: what medical school the doctor went to, in what areas he or she specializes and whether the doctor is board-certified (which means he or she passed advanced, qualifying exams in his or her specialty). Ask if the doctor is associated with a teaching hospital, which is usually a guarantee that the doctor's training is very up-to-date.

The ob-gyn I eventually chose was well qualified and connected with one of the best hospitals in the D.C. area. Most important, he had a sweet, gentle manner and made me instantly comfortable. A good doctor should relate to you as a person and ask questions about your lifestyle and any emotional issues that might be relevant to get a complete picture. The doctor shouldn't make you feel rushed when you are speaking.

It may not be practical to pre-interview a doctor, so you may not discover until after a first visit whether you find him or her compatible. Bottom line: Use common sense and follow your instincts. If you feel unsure about a doctor, find another one. It is important to be very candid when you are a patient, and you may not be inclined to do that with someone who doesn't make you comfortable. Worse, a distant and unempathic doctor may make you even more anxious than you would ordinarily be. And although warmth and kindness are no guarantee of a doctor's competence, it stands to reason that someone who cares about people will take more interest in every case.

I find that people who are very selective about a hairdresser or an auto mechanic are willing to put up with medical care from someone they don't necessarily like and haven't checked out thoroughly. That doesn't make sense.

Make the most of each visit. Visiting the doctor is an anxiety-producing experience for many people, but it's like cleaning up your files or similar good-for-you responsibilities. Once it's over, you'll feel terrific. Make the most of the visit by planning for it. Don't keep your concerns from your doctor. Before the visit, make a list of anything that's troubling you— headaches, stomach upsets, rashes, whatever—and jot down the details that the doctor will want to know: dates of each occurrence, frequency and any other fact that may shed light on the problem, such as what you were eating before a symptom arose. Write down any questions you may have. And take notes when the doctor gives you answers and instructions. It's amazing how easily you can forget what the doctor said to do, particularly if you're a little nervous. Keep those notes for your medical history book (see page 218). If the problem recurs—"Didn't I have that rash before? What cream did I use?"—it will be very useful to have a record. (This is handy advice for moms, too. Not only is it hard to recall details, it's amazing how you can forget which kid had what ailment when.)

Be totally open. Don't hold back your concerns or questions about intimate problems or be afraid to reveal that you smoke or drink. Physicians aren't there to judge you but to help you. Conditions that you may find embarrassing, such as pain during intercourse or urinary incontinence, can often be easily treated or can at least shed light on your medical condition.

Get involved in the process. If you have, or suspect you may have, a particular illness, read about it so you know what questions to ask your doctor. Many health newsletters, books, magazines and Web sites can enhance your understanding of current medical practice. If you see contradictory information, talk things over with your doctor. Your informed point of view will help ensure that you get the best possible treatment.

Keep track of your family medical history. Keep a medical "résumé" of your family's history as well as your own illnesses, injuries, hospitalizations and surgeries from childhood to the present. Keep other medical information, such as notes you take after doctors' visits and any X-ray films that you are given to keep, in the same place.

If you switch doctors, get a copy of your records for your new doctor and another copy for your home medical file.

Heart disease, breast cancer, thyroid disease, glaucoma, osteoporosis and other diseases often have genetic links. Knowing your family health history may help your doctor to be alert for, diagnose and perhaps prevent and/or cure whatever may ail you, and records of your own health history can help your doctor make a diagnosis or decide what tests to order. These can be vital in the event of an emergency.

They can also spare you a lot of anxiety. I went to donate blood one day but was told, "You can't. Your iron is low. You're on the borderline." I was just devastated! When I called the internist who tests me regularly, he told me to relax. "Denise, that's your normal reading. You've been like this for years, and I can assure you you're not anemic." That was such an enormous relief. You need records of all your baseline medical tests—from blood tests to X rays.

Make copies of the following forms for yourself (and, if you're inclined, for other family members, too). Use this to help keep a record of when a checkup is due. Add pages as needed to keep track of any other tests or checkups, and keep your records up to date.

TEN MUST-HAVE MEDICAL TESTS

Early detection is key to overcoming many serious diseases. Most people know this, but they still don't get important medical tests because they're afraid of what the doctors may find. What's scarier is thinking about what the doctors *don't* find. Discovering any illness before you have symptoms may buy you valuable treatment time. Following are 10 key tests that you should get or consider annually (unless your doctor tells you otherwise), particularly after you've reached the big four-oh.

Family History

Mother	Father
Age at death: _____	Age at death: _____
Cause of death: _____	Cause of death: _____
Significant illnesses: _____	Significant illnesses: _____
_____	_____
_____	_____

Sibling(s)	Sibling(s)
Age at death: _____	Age at death: _____
Cause of death: _____	Cause of death: _____
Significant illnesses: _____	Significant illnesses: _____
_____	_____
_____	_____

Sibling(s)	Sibling(s)
Age at death: _____	Age at death: _____
Cause of death: _____	Cause of death: _____
Significant illnesses: _____	Significant illnesses: _____
_____	_____
_____	_____

Aunt(s)	Aunt(s)
Age at death: _____	Age at death: _____
Cause of death: _____	Cause of death: _____
Significant illnesses: _____	Significant illnesses: _____
_____	_____
_____	_____

Uncle(s)	Uncle(s)
Age at death: _____	Age at death: _____
Cause of death: _____	Cause of death: _____
Significant illnesses: _____	Significant illnesses: _____
_____	_____
_____	_____

Maternal grandmother	Maternal grandfather
Age at death: _____	Age at death: _____
Cause of death: _____	Cause of death: _____
Significant illnesses: _____	Significant illnesses: _____
_____	_____
_____	_____

Paternal grandmother	Paternal grandfather
Age at death: _____	Age at death: _____
Cause of death: _____	Cause of death: _____
Significant illnesses: _____	Significant illnesses: _____
_____	_____
_____	_____

Personal History

Vaccinations	Type	Date	
Current Medications	Type	Dosage	Frequency
Allergies	Type	Treatment	

Do you currently smoke?

If so, _____ cigarettes a day.

If not, did you ever smoke?

How long?

When did you stop?

How many drinks do you have per day? _____ per week? _____

Pregnancies (dates) _____

_____

Live births (dates and vaginal/C-section) _____

_____

Have you had chicken pox _____(date), mumps _____(date),
measles _____(date)?

Record of Illnesses and Injuries

Illnesses	Type	Date	Details
Injuries			
Hospitalizations			
Surgeries			

Record of Checkups

	Doctor	Date	Date	Date	Date
Blood tests					
Pap smear/ breast exam					
Mammography					
Colorectal					
Colonoscopy					
Bone density					
Dermatological					
Eye					
Periodontal					
Dental					

Type of Test	Date	Result	Date	Result	Date	Result	Date	Result
Total cholesterol								
HDL								
LDL								
Triglycerides								
Blood glucose								

1. Blood Pressure

Cardiovascular disease, I was surprised to discover, is the number-one cause of death for women as well as men. One of the reasons it's so dangerous is that in women there are often few if any outward symptoms. But this disease *can* be diagnosed in routine tests. You probably didn't give any thought to your blood pressure readings in your 20s and 30s. But you need to pay more attention to those numbers as you age. Most annual physicals include a blood pressure check. The top reading (systolic pressure) measures pressure when the heart is contracting, and the bottom reading (diastolic pressure) measures pressure when your heart is relaxed. The doctor looks at both. A normal range for systolic pressure is 100 to 140; for diastolic it's 60 to 90. Readings of 140 to 159 (systolic) and/or 90 to 94 (diastolic) are considered mild hypertension.

According to the American Heart Association, high blood pressure is a risk factor for both heart attacks and strokes. If you do have high blood pressure, your doctor can prescribe drugs to bring it down to a safer level. Regular exercise, weight loss and a diet rich in fresh fruit and veggies and low in sodium and red meat can also help bring blood pressure down.

2. Cholesterol

High cholesterol is another major risk factor for heart disease and stroke. Cholesterol is a soft, waxy substance that builds up in your blood and has been linked to the formation of plaque. Plaque blocks your arteries, preventing adequate quantities of blood from passing through. Even women who eat healthy, low-fat diets and exercise regularly may have a genetic predisposition to high cholesterol. The only way to know what's going on in your body is through a blood test. Most doctors order a cholesterol screening as part of an annual checkup.

There are two main types of cholesterol. LDL cholesterol is the "bad" kind that sticks to the arterial walls, where it contributes to the buildup of plaque. HDL cholesterol is the "good" kind that carries the LDL out of your body. In addition to those numbers, the lab should report your total cholesterol level.

A total cholesterol level of less than 200 is considered desirable; it indicates that you are at low risk for cardiovascular disease. But even if your total cholesterol is borderline high (between 200 and 239), you should be okay if your HDL is also high (35 or above). If not, your doctor may prescribe cholesterol-lowering drugs.

A blood test may also check your level of triglycerides, a type of fat

What Cholesterol Level Should You Be Aiming For?

Total cholesterol
Desirable (low risk): less than 200
Borderline high risk: 200–239
High risk: 240 or higher

LDL ("bad" cholesterol)
Desirable (low risk): less than 130
Borderline high risk: 130–159
High risk: 160 or higher

HDL ("good" cholesterol)
Desirable (low risk): 35 or higher
High risk: less than 35

Source: American Heart Association

that circulates in your blood. If you have high blood cholesterol as well as high triglycerides, your risk for heart disease is probably greater than if you only had high triglycerides. A normal reading is between 10 and 250, but your triglyceride level may be too high if it's above 150, depending on what other risk factors you have for heart disease

If you do have elevated cholesterol, whether or not you are put on medication you should be careful about consuming foods high in saturated fat and cholesterol. For the most part, these are high-fat animal products such as red meat, butter, eggs, cream and some fried foods. Instead, try to eat foods high in fiber such as vegetables and high-fiber breads, red grapes, and low-fat soy foods, all of which should help reduce cholesterol and may also help raise your HDL level. And if you haven't already, lose weight, stop smoking and start exercising regularly.

3. Blood Sugar/Glucose

Diabetes ranks as the fourth-leading killer among diseases in the United States. It occurs when your body doesn't produce enough insulin, the hormone needed to convert sugar into energy.

There are two types of diabetes. Type 1 is usually diagnosed during childhood, but type 2 tends to occur primarily in adults who are over 40. Warning signs include cuts that are slow to heal, tingling in the hands and feet, chronic skin, gum and bladder infections—and, most commonly, constant thirst and frequent urination. Despite these warnings, less than half of adult diabetics are aware they are ill. That's why it's important that your doctor includes a blood test for elevated blood sugar or glucose levels in your annual physical, especially if you're over 40, are overweight or have a family history of diabetes.

Many diabetes sufferers can control the disease by changing their diets or taking drugs designed to stabilize their blood sugar. When diabetes isn't managed properly, the result can be anything from a heart attack or a stroke to kidney failure, amputation or blindness.

For every 2.2 pounds of extra weight, the risk of diabetes increases 4.5 percent. Overall, the number of diabetics increased 33 percent from 1990 to 1998, with the disease affecting 6.5 percent of the population by the end of that period, compared to 4.9 percent at the beginning of the decade, a recent study in the journal *Diabetes Care* reported. Diabetes may be on the rise because more people are gaining weight and not getting enough exercise. But you won't be one of them, will you?

4. Pap Smear

Having an annual Pap smear so that a laboratory can examine cells from your cervix is your best defense against cervical cancer. Many cases of this disease are linked to the human papilloma virus (HPV), a sexually transmitted virus that doesn't always have visible symptoms and may go undetected for years. An estimated 80 percent of Americans are infected. If either you or your mate has ever been with another partner, you may have the virus. Even if you don't have HPV, you may be at risk for cervical cancer as you get older.

The good news is that Pap smears detect up to 90 percent of cases before symptoms develop, while the cancer is still treatable. The Food and Drug Administration recently approved three new techniques to screen for cervical cancer. AutoPap and PapNet are computerized systems that evaluate Pap slides. ThinPrep is a way of preparing samples to be viewed by laboratory technicians. Talk to your doctor about whether to consider any of these.

After three or more consecutive Pap smears with normal results, your doctor may recommend less frequent testing.

If you are experiencing any sort of gynecological problem or discomfort, call your physician right away. Don't wait and worry until your next exam to find out if what's happening is normal. Pain during and between periods, irregular or heavy bleeding, abdominal pain, unusual discharge, excessive bloating or a feeling of pressure in the lower abdomen may indicate a gynecological problem, including a sexually transmitted disease, endometriosis or ovarian cancer. But they also may indicate a relatively innocuous bacterial infection. Do yourself a favor and find out.

5. Colorectal Cancer

This is another disease that is often thought of as primarily a male problem. Not true. Colorectal cancer is the third-leading cause of cancer death among American women. Like many types of cancer, it is highly treatable if caught early, but there aren't always early symptoms. As a result, less than half of those who have it are diagnosed before the disease has spread.

That's why routine early screenings are essential. If you have a personal or family history of colorectal cancer, polyps or inflammatory bowel disease, your doctor may recommend you start a screening program at age 40 or even earlier. But for most people, the American Cancer Society recommends that screenings begin at age 40. Regular testing should include a yearly fecal occult blood test (FOBT) that is performed by a laboratory using a stool sample. In addition, you should have a flexible sigmoidoscopy every five years and a colonoscopy every ten.

In a sigmoidoscopy or colonoscopy, a specialist (a gastroenterologist or a proctologist) checks the interior of the colon. The doctor checks only the lower portion of the large bowel in the former procedure but the entire colon in the latter. In the course of the examination, the doctor may discover and remove polyps, abnormal growths that usually start to form in the midlife years and that may or may not be precancerous. Many people are very fearful of this procedure, but most experience little or no discomfort, since you are medicated to feel relaxed and drowsy.

If you experience rectal bleeding, a change in your bowel habits, unexplained weight loss and/or abdominal or back pain, contact a physician right away. You may not be seriously ill. However, if a problem exists, you may be saving your own life. In addition to getting regular exams, you can cut your colon cancer risk by—you've heard it before—engaging in regular exercise, maintaining a good weight and eating a healthy diet. Although recent research doesn't support the long-held notion that a high-fiber diet cuts the risk of colon cancer in particular, a healthy diet is known to cut cancer risk in general.

6. Breast Cancer

At age 40 your risk for this disease is 1 in 217. By 45 it's 1 in 93. The majority of women who get breast cancer are in their 50s and 60s.

As with other types of cancer, early detection is crucial. In some women a lump can be felt, but in others there is no warning signs. Only 6 percent of breast cancer cases start with pain. Most women find tumors themselves, so monthly self-exams are critical. Getting into the habit of doing those exams helps you notice even small changes in your breast tissue and also teaches you to recognize normal irregularities in your own breast and distinguish them from something new and suspicious.

During your yearly checkup, your ob-gyn will usually perform a manual breast exam. Recent studies indicate that the manual exam alone can be highly effective in detecting and preventing fatalities from this disease, but now that you're over 40, you should also be getting annual mammograms. Mammograms may detect tiny lumps that can't be felt by either you or your doctor. If your doctor doesn't talk to you about getting one, be sure to ask. Many insurance plans and HMOs will cover the cost; if yours doesn't, call the American Cancer Society (800-ACS-2345) for local resource information.

Since going for a mammogram is such a source of anxiety, I will pass on to you a wonderful idea. A group of women I know plan a yearly event around getting their mammograms together. If everything is fine, and so far it has been, they go out to celebrate. Most important, since they have put this day aside, they never cancel or postpone their tests.

If you find a lump or one shows up on a mammogram, don't panic immediately. The majority of breast lumps turn out to be harmless. Many are benign, fluid-filled cysts that can be easily drained. (Benign cysts are the most common cause of lumps in women ages 30 to 50.) Still, you should let your doctor know immediately about anything that seems suspicious. Depending on your health history, the doctor may tell you to wait a month or two to see if the lump goes away, and then, if it hasn't, to go for further testing.

Even if there is no lump you can feel, a tumor may change the breast in ways you can see. Be sure to call your doctor if you notice any of the following:

- An increase in the size or number of veins in part or all of one breast
- A nipple that points in a different direction than it used to
- A dimpled area on the breast where the skin is pulling in
- Redness or a prominent pore in the breast skin
- A shape change, such as a bulge or dip
- A rash or eczema-like patch on the breast, or a sore on a nipple
- Nipple discharge

A great deal of research is going on in breast cancer. Short-term studies involving more than 12,000 women have shown that a new osteoporosis medication, raloxifene (trade name Evista) may prevent breast cancer in healthy postmenopausal women. This FDA-approved drug was associated with a 62 percent reduction in new breast cancer cases when used over a period of one month to nearly three years. Being marketed as an alternative to estrogen replacement therapy (ERT), the drug has a few side effects, including hot flashes and leg cramps, and also may be associated with a risk of blood clots. If you believe you might benefit from raloxifene, consult your doctor.

7. Skin Cancer

Despite all that time spent in the sun as a kid, I've been lucky. No suspicious moles or growths have turned up so far. But people like me who've had a lot of sun exposure should see a dermatologist for a head-to-toe skin exam once a year. Melanoma, the most serious form of skin cancer, is on the rise in the United States. In the last 25 years the number of cases has more than doubled.

At the doctor's office melanoma checks are usually done visually. There is also a technique called "mole mapping," in which skin discolorations are scanned and recorded into a computer; at your next visit another scan is taken, then the images are compared to see what changes have occurred.

Aside from your annual date with a dermatologist, you should check your own skin for irregularities regularly. I try to do a full once-over each month. To remember what to look for, think ABCD. That's a memory device to alert you that you are looking for any freckles or moles

- that are *a*symmetrical, meaning the shape of one half doesn't match the shape of the other
- that have an irregular *b*order or pigment that spreads into the surrounding skin
- that are uneven in *c*olor
- that are large in *d*iameter, usually bigger than a pencil eraser

If you notice any such thing, call a doctor right away.

8. Eyesight

Have you noticed that your arms seem to be growing shorter now that you're 40? You can't hold the phone book far enough away to get it into focus. You don't need a bone doctor, you need an eye doctor. If you always had good vision but now have trouble doing close work or your eyes feel tired or weak because of eyestrain, you may need reading glasses.

Health: Body Sense for Women

Even if you don't need glasses or have any acute symptom such as sudden vision changes in one or both eyes, unexplainable and lasting redness or ongoing eye pain, you should still have a complete eye exam every two or three years and yearly after age 50. This is very important if you have a family history of problems like glaucoma, a progressive disease that may result in blindness. Glaucoma occurs when pressure builds up inside the eye, causing damage to eye nerves. It doesn't always cause early symptoms but is easily detected during a routine eye exam by a painless test that measures the pressure of fluid inside your eye. If caught early, the disease is easily treated.

During a routine eye exam the doctor will also look inside your eye with specialized equipment that can diagnose medical conditions such as diabetes and hypertension along with a variety of specific eye disorders such as cataracts. Cataracts occur when protein buildup causes the lenses of your eyes to become cloudy. In most cases cataracts occur in people over 65. You may be able to prevent this problem in the future by wearing sunglasses regularly and eating a diet high in antioxidants.

9. Bone Density

One out of four American women is losing bone at a dangerously accelerated rate. About 25 percent of women over 60 have osteoporosis, a condition that can result in fragile bones and a hunched-over posture. A lack of sufficient calcium in your diet increases your risk, as do several other factors, including drinking and smoking, a family history of the disease, a small frame, and exercise so excessively strenuous that it stops your menstrual periods. Ask your gynecologist or internist at what age you should start to be screened for osteoporosis via a bone density test.

The most accurate tests involve low-dose X rays of your spine and hip to measure the mineral content of the bone. (Bone spurs associated with aging may make a diagnosis of spine and hip pictures difficult, so your forearm may be X-rayed as well.)

If your bones aren't dense enough, you'll be told to increase your intake of calcium and vitamin D, engage in weight-bearing exercise, stop smoking and cut back on alcohol intake. Estrogen or hormone replacement therapy (ERT or HRT) can help slow bone loss, but there may be risks involved with taking hormones. (See page 234.) Other remedies for bone loss include daily doses of a bisphosphonate (a drug that increases bone mineral density and reduces bone loss) or calcitonin (a hormone that helps to prevent bone loss). Researchers are working on new drugs to reverse the process of bone loss.

10. Teeth and Gums

When I was very little I brushed my teeth so I wouldn't have cavities. When I was a teenager I worried not just about cavities, but also about— good heavens!—bad breath. Nowadays I'm also thinking about gum disease, which occurs when plaque (caused by bacteria) causes gum tissue to pull away from the teeth. Left untreated, the tissue of the gums can become loose enough to cause tooth loss.

To keep plaque under control, you need periodic professional examinations and cleaning. If you start out with a good, clean mouth, it's easier to do cleanings at home. Get to a hygienist every six months, and follow up with careful brushing and flossing daily. Most of us need to be shown how to brush properly and thoroughly. So brush up on your brushing technique at the checkup. Ask your dentist or hygienist to recommend techniques and suggest products that would be helpful—not just toothbrushes, floss and toothpaste, but also gum stimulators and over-the-counter dental disclosing agents that show you where plaque exists.

FIVE OTHER HEALTH CONCERNS AFTER FORTY

Your family history, your lifestyle or any unusual symptoms may mean that you need to talk to your doctor about one or more of the following:

1. Thyroid Malfunction

The thyroid gland, located inside the neck, is a very influential little organ. It releases two hormones that control heart rate, body temperature and the speed with which the body burns calories. These hormones also affect strength, appetite, mood, brain function and skin and hair texture.

Some 13 million Americans—most of them women—suffer from an over- or underactive thyroid. And because this gland has so much responsibility, it can create a whole slew of problems if it's not working right. Hypothyroidism, or an underactive thyroid, can cause fatigue, memory loss and sudden weight gain and may create what appears to be psychologically caused depression. Untreated, it can also raise cholesterol levels.

Hyperthyroidism, an overactive thyroid, puts the body in overdrive. Symptoms include a racing heart, anxiety, heart arrhythmia, weight loss, bone loss and muscle weakness. Women with hyperthyroidism may also have sleep problems.

Since many of these symptoms are subtle and can mimic other problems, thyroid problems often go undiagnosed. Fortunately, new blood tests can detect the slightest rise or dip in hormone levels, and anyone with a family history of thyroid problems should be tested. Ask your doctor if you should have your thyroid checked if you are experiencing any unusual symptoms.

2. Varicose Veins

Starting in your 40s, you may begin to discover little purple or red squiggles, like a spiderweb, on your ankles or legs. These spider veins, as they are called, are like the teasers for varicose veins, which are the main event. Both are caused by the same factors and both can occur anywhere on the body but usually show up on the legs.

In healthy veins blood travels toward the heart, helped by resilient vein walls and one-way valves that combat gravity's downward pull. But defective valves or a weakness in the vein walls sometimes allows blood to flow backward and pool in the vein so it bulges under the skin, creating a ropelike pattern.

Spider veins may cause dull aches. Varicose veins typically cause tired, achy and heavy-feeling legs and, in some cases, night cramps.

No one really knows what causes varicose veins, but there seems to be some congenital link and also some connection to female hormones. Women have varicose veins three times as often as men, frequently linked to pregnancy or the use of birth control pills.

A problem with varicose veins is progressive, and they can't be prevented, but you can minimize their effects in the following ways:

- Try not to stand in one place for longer than 15 minutes.
- Avoid sitting for more than 30 minutes at a time.
- Do not wear socks or stockings that leave marks on the leg (such as knee-highs that leave an indentation).
- If you have a family history of varicose veins and/or you stand a lot at work, wear support hose with graduated compression (tightest at the ankle). Many brands are available without a prescription (in styles for both men and women), such as Jobst, Juzo, Sigvaris, Venosan and Medi.
- Wear support socks or hose when flying, when visiting a high altitude and during the second and third trimesters of pregnancy.
- Exercise such as walking and bicycling helps to develop the pumping action of the calf muscles and boost circulation in the legs.

- Avoid exercises that cause sudden, prolonged muscle contraction, such as heavy weight lifting with the legs. Instead, do exercises that involve more repetition with less weight.
- If you notice swollen ankles, sleep with your legs up on a pillow, higher than your heart.
- Maintain a healthy weight.

Varicose veins occasionally cause serious complications. These include leg swelling and phlebitis (inflammation and clotting), which can be disabling and painful. On rare occasions blood clots that occur in varicose veins can dislodge and travel to the lungs. Sudden pain, redness, swelling or warmth of the leg should be reported to your doctor immediately.

The standard procedure for removing large varicose veins in the past was vein stripping, which involves tying off the ends of the vein and removing it through an incision in the groin. But in a new, less invasive technique called closure, a catheter is inserted into a tiny incision behind or on the side of the knee and then worked into the vein. Radio-frequency energy heats the vein from the inside, sealing it shut. Vein stripping involves a large scar and a week-long recovery, but most patients can resume normal activity immediately after closure, which leaves only a tiny nick. Closure has a success rate of 95 percent, just like vein stripping, but it was approved by the FDA in 1999 and is not yet widely utilized. Ask your doctor if you might be a candidate.

3. Ovarian Cancer

This silent killer claimed the lives of courageous *Harper's Bazaar* editor Liz Tilberis and of a former exercise client and friend of mine, the wonderful comedienne Gilda Radner.

There is no infallible test for ovarian cancer, and the warning signs are subtle, partially because the ovaries are located so deep inside the pelvis. Usually this cancer is detected only after a surgical examination and a biopsy, at which point it may have already spread. Only 25 percent of cases are discovered in stage I, when it is confined to one or both ovaries.

However, at age 40 the likelihood of your getting ovarian cancer is only 15.7 per 100,000. The risk increases when you're over 60, rising to 54 per 100,000 at age 79.

You are at higher risk if a member of your immediate family (mother, sister and/or daughter) has been diagnosed with the disease; if you have a personal history of breast cancer or the genetic markers for breast and ovarian cancer; if you are of Ashkenazi Jewish descent and have a genetic marker; and/or if you've never been pregnant. Be alert to the warning symptoms. If one or more of these persists for a month, see your doctor:

- Vague, chronic gastrointestinal discomfort, such as gas, nausea or indigestion
- Frequent and/or urgent need to urinate
- Change in bowel habits
- Abnormal vaginal bleeding
- Pelvic or abdominal swelling that may or may not be accompanied by pain
- Loss of appetite or feeling full even after the lightest meal
- Unexplained fatigue
- Shortness of breath
- Pain during intercourse

A new blood test for CA-125 can detect the presence of proteins shed by some cancer cells. It may be able to detect a recurrence of the disease in women who have already been treated.

More than 25,000 American women will be diagnosed with ovarian cancer this year. Thanks to new drugs and treatments, over the past 30 years, the survival rate has doubled.

4. HIV/AIDS

AIDS remains the leading cause of death for women in the United States between the ages of 25 and 44, according to the Centers for Disease Control and Prevention. The number of AIDS cases reported among adult women has more than tripled in the past decade. You should not have sex with a new partner until you have both been tested. If, however, you have ever had unprotected sex with a partner whose sexual history you do not know, you should take an HIV test.

New, FDA-approved at-home tests can be ordered on the Web at www.homeaccess.com. At press time, the test cost $55 and takes three business days to get the results.

5. Sex After 40

Do not think that age is the barometer for what your sex life will be like down the road. *The Starr-Weiner Report on Sex and Sexuality in the Mature Years* (1981) and E. Brecher's *Love, Sex, and Aging* (1984) are among the works that have confirmed that the need and desire for sex continues indefinitely and that if a partner is available, regular sexual activity is typical. A MacArthur Foundation study indicated that while the frequency of sex does decline with age, men and women ages 45 to 54 rated their sex lives and relationships "excellent." Many of them reported enjoying sex more than people half their age and declared themselves to be more satisfied with their partners than they were ten years ago.

Many women find that their 40s are a time of increased sexual satisfaction. At this point you are more comfortable with your body and your sexuality than when you were younger. Intimacy with a partner is often more fulfilling, and reaching orgasm may become easier. And if you're like many women who've turned to exercise in the past decade or so, you may be as physically fit as ever—or perhaps even more so.

Isn't that great? I think sex is an important part of a loving relationship, and certainly it should be part of any healthy woman's life.

LOOKING TO THE DECADE AHEAD

Menopause

When I turned 40 I found myself watching for signs of menopause. Is my period tapering off or am I just having a light cycle? Am I being uncharacteristically short-tempered or crabby? Are those hot flashes or is the room just exceptionally hot? If you're like me, you're unsure of what to expect and nervous about how it will feel.

For most 40-year-olds, menopause is still down the road a piece. Though some women become menopausal as young as 35, the average woman in this country reaches menopause at 51, though no one can predict exactly when it will happen. There is no correlation between the age at which you start your period and the age you reach menopause, or between menopause and your race, height, number of children you have or whether or not you took birth control pills. There may be some correlation with the age your mother was at when she achieved menopause, and it appears that smokers and former smokers can reach menopause two years earlier than nonsmokers.

What we call menopause is in fact several different stages. The earliest is perimenopause, which usually begins in your late 40s and lasts several years. This is when symptoms begin: irregular periods, spotting, night sweats and/or hot flashes.

Technically, menopause is the moment in time when your ovaries run out of eggs. Every woman starts out with a lifetime's supply, and then over the years she runs out. (A science writer and friend of mine once compared a woman's ovaries to a huge gumball machine that gets depleted over time.) At menopause, your period stops for good.

But wait until you've gone full a 12 months without a period before you throw out the tampons and stop using birth control—unless you like surprises that need diapering.

This period, from perimenopause through permanent cessation of menstrual periods, lasts for years—years that for some women become an emotional roller coaster, as they feel alternately moody, sad or out of control. These unpredictable emotions occur because when you run out of eggs, you also stop producing the sex hormones estrogen, progesterone and testosterone. Many women also suffer unsettling physical side effects such as hot flashes, fatigue, vaginal dryness or difficulty sleeping.

The good news? According to the MacArthur Foundation study, women who had already gone through menopause said its emotional and physical effects were overemphasized in the popular media and culture. In fact, 62 percent of postmenopausal women reported "only relief" and a mere 2 percent reported "regret."

My mother had a very easy menopause and never reported any unsettling side effects or symptoms. Many of my friends going through menopause are relatively free of problems. I personally don't have many concerns. I certainly won't miss having a period. And I think one of the reasons so many women in the past had a difficult time is that menopause marked the end of their ability to reproduce, which at one time very much defined who women were.

But my friends and I and the other women I know have managed to "get a life" that isn't defined simply by others—by our home, mothering and marriage. Even if menopause occurs simultaneously with an empty nest and a husband's midlife crisis (another reason it may have been so devastating), we have many plans for the postmenopausal part of our lives. We aren't feeling sad, we are feeling optimistic and we are determined to keep ourselves healthy and happy.

To Hormone or Not to Hormone During your perimenopausal years, discuss any unusual symptoms, either physical or emotional, with a health care professional. These may indicate some other, unrelated problem, or they may indeed be side effects of menopause. Sleep problems, for example, are often menopause-related. So are changes in your libido and also vaginal dryness, which may cause discomfort during intercourse. The dryness may be relieved with a water-based lubricant such as K-Y jelly. Evening primrose oil may help with hot flashes. Or you may want to consider hormone replacement therapy (HRT). There are pros and cons to this choice.

On the good side, HRT may prevent heart disease over the long term by lowering LDL ("bad" cholesterol) levels and keeping blood vessels healthy. It probably protects against osteoporosis by keeping calcium from leaching out of your bones. Researchers at Indiana University may have found a link between lowered estrogen levels and cataracts. There is also some speculation that estrogen replacement can delay the onset of Alzheimer's disease and improve memory.

On the other hand, to protect your heart and bones you must continue taking hormones for the rest of your life. And HRT may increase your risk of uterine cancer, breast cancer, gallbladder disease, blood clots, diabetes and severe high blood pressure. Despite years of research, there is no definitive answer to the question of whether or not you should go for it.

Before you decide, you and a doctor should review your medical history, taking into account your personal and family history of heart disease, breast cancer, breast lumps, osteoporosis, abnormal vaginal bleeding and abnormal blood clotting. The age at which you delivered

Frequently Asked Questions About Hormone Replacement Therapy

Will HRT make me fat?

According to the North American Menopause Society, there's no link between either menopause or HRT and weight gain. Some women taking hormones may find that progesterone causes them to retain water, but the changes on the scale should be very slight. Any real gains are more likely due to a slowing metabolism, inactivity or overeating. Major shifts in your weight should always be discussed with your physician.

Are "natural" hormones safer than the kinds my doctor prescribes?

Experts say no. There is only one kind of "natural" hormone, and that's the kind your own body makes. While prescription HRT has been highly researched and tested, many over-the-counter remedies—the kind you find in health food stores and drugstores—have not been well studied and aren't regulated by any government agency. Talk to your doctor before you start self-medicating with any drug, herb or supplement. Some herbs are known to interfere with certain drugs, which could lead to a dangerous interaction.

Soy products—milk, soy nuts, boiled soybeans and tofu—reduce LDL cholesterol. Since there was a suggestion that soy also reduced hot flashes and the risk of breast cancer, some women have been taking soy supplements instead of estrogen. But testing has shown soy may have no impact on hot flashes. More troubling, in the women who took soy supplements (between 38 and 45 mg of soy isoflavones in the form of a fortified powder or protein beverage) there was a proliferation of breast cells that might increase their risk of breast cancer. Until more tests are done, stick to moderate amounts (4 to 5 ounces) of whole soy foods.

Keeping Cool Through Hot Flashes

- If you're standing up or exercising, find a place to sit and breathe deeply until the flash passes.

- Dress in layers (so you can peel off clothing when temps hit the roof).

- Drink plenty of water, herbal tea and other noncaffeinated liquids.

- Don't smoke.

- Eliminate or cut back on caffeine, alcohol, sugar and spicy foods.

- Get regular massages or meditate to keep stress levels in check.

- Buy yourself one of those personal fans—and don't be embarrassed to use it! Heck, everybody interesting has an unusual habit.

your first child and the severity of your menopausal side effects also may factor into your decision.

No matter what you decide, you can minimize your discomfort and improve your long-term health outlook by making positive lifestyle changes—which would include basically everything that we've been talking about in this book! Life really can begin again at 40. Now's the time to make that decision to stop smoking, watch your weight, exercise and eat a healthy diet.

Finding the Support Group You Need A friend of mine recently went to the supermarket, shopped, loaded the groceries into the cart, wheeled the cart to the curb, got into her car and drove directly home. Only when she pulled into her driveway and looked in the (empty) backseat did she realize what she had done. Believe me, you'll probably have one or more "menopausal moments" of your own, when you can't recall a friend's phone number, you look for your glasses for an hour only to discover them on your head, or pull the refrigerator door open and then can't remember why you're there.

Some women joke about these moments, but others have a harder time dealing with them. What seems to be really helpful for many people is reading about menopause online or reaching to others for support. When in doubt, talk it out. It's a big help to share the issues of our own forgetful 40s and 50s just the way we helped one another cope with our kids' terrible twos. Two excellent menopause Web sites are the North American Menopause Society's site (www.menopause.org) and that of Power Surge (www.powersurge.com).

Protecting Your Ticker

Heart disease? That's a guy thing, isn't it? The answer is no. Heart disease is the number-one cause of death among American women. But there is a great deal that you can do to protect yourself against this problem.

Your risk of heart disease increases significantly after menopause unless you're on HRT, because at that point most women don't have adequate levels of estrogen, which helps keep your blood cholesterol levels down and your blood vessels elastic. Though your hormone levels drop, unfortunately your craving for french fries and bacon cheeseburgers and pepperoni pizza may not. And the snacking may eventually result in weight gain.

Extra weight, of course, increases your risk for heart disease, but in addition a decline in estrogen means the fat you put on is more likely to accumulate around your abdomen than on your hips and thighs. You may be getting a tummy for the first time. Carrying weight in your stomach is bad healthwise, because "apple shapes" are at higher risk of cardiovascular disease than pear shapes. If you want to calculate your waist-to-hip ratio (WHR), use a tape measure to measure first the smallest part of your waist and then the largest part of your hips and buttocks. Divide your waist measurement by your hip measurement. For example, if your waist measures 30 inches and your hips are 38 inches, the ratio is approximately .79. This is your waist-to-hip ratio. In general, women with a ratio higher than .85 are at high risk for heart disease. If you're between .80 and .85, you're at moderate risk. If you're below .80, you're at low risk. Even if your WHR is A-okay, it's wise to

New Developments in Heart Disease Research

In recent years scientists have identified a strong link between heart disease and high blood levels of the amino acid homocysteine. Homocysteine buildup can be prevented by cutting back on animal products (fatty meat, eggs, butter) and sugary, processed foods (donuts, candy, cookies) as well as consuming more B vitamins and folic acid (folate). (See "Supplemental Knowledge" on pages 136–43.) Also note in Chapter 4 that some studies suggest that vitamin E may help prevent the buildup of fatty plaque on artery walls.

While aspirin isn't routinely recommended for prevention of heart attacks and strokes, numerous studies have shown it to be beneficial for people with prior histories of cardiovascular disease. The popular painkiller can help inhibit dangerous arterial clots. Some doctors have even recommended taking an aspirin or letting one dissolve under your tongue if you have any sudden chest pain. If you have narrowing of the arteries, the American Heart Association recommends taking one baby aspirin (81 mg) a day, but since aspirin may cause gastrointestinal problems, consult your doctor first.

take a few steps to keep heart disease risk low by eating right, exercising regularly and not smoking.

What's very important for you to know about heart disease is that the symptoms are very different for women than for men. While men most typically have a heart attack that is a dramatic event—the kind you see in the movies, where people clutch at their chests—women instead tend to have milder and chronic symptoms like fatigue and shortness of breath, not necessarily after exertion but from time to time, and even in the middle of the night. They may feel a dull, achy discomfort rather than a sharp pain. Often women will have symptoms that they interpret as gastrointestinal problems rather than heart issues, and they may even have pain or pressure radiating into the jaw or neck. Both women and men may have pain in the left arm or elbow, dizziness, or light-headedness. Because these symptoms are so nonspecific, many women are not properly diagnosed for heart disease. Be sure to mention any symptoms like these to your doctor.

Tightening Up the Pelvic Muscles

Women may have feelings of weakness in the pelvis after childbirth or due to hormonal changes related to pregnancy or menopause. The common cause is prolapsed uterus, a stretching of the ligaments and tissues that normally keep the womb in place. One result may be stress incontinence—that involuntary trickle of urine that comes when you laugh, cough, sneeze or strain. Another may be that during intercourse, the muscles of the vagina don't seem as "tight" to your partner.

Any such problem should be reported to your doctor, who may prescribe some other form of medication or recommend surgery. One simple way to reduce the problem is to avoid bladder irritants and diuretics such as artificial sweeteners, fruit juices, alcohol, carbonated beverages, coffee, tea and other caffeinated drinks. If the problem is mild, the solution is often Kegel exercises.

With the easy-to-do Kegel exercises, you may be able to prevent this problem before it arises or get relief once it exists. Sixty percent of women who do Kegels report significant improvement and 15 to 20 percent return to normal bladder function.

Breathe Your Way to Better Health

If there's one thing you probably thought you were doing right, it's breathing. But there's a way to do it better. As you breathe, you pump oxygen to all the cells and muscles of your body. The deeper you breathe, the more oxygen you take in, whether you're walking on a treadmill or

How to Do a Kegel

For best results, do these for two minutes two to three times a day and prior to or during any activity that usually causes leakage. Remember: To strengthen your pelvic floor muscles, you must work them harder than they're used to. If you continue challenging them, you should see a change in as little as three to four weeks.

Ready to get cracking on those Kegels? Let's go.

Step 1: Find Your Target Muscles

These muscles are a lot harder to locate than your biceps! You'll need a little practice.

1. Sit or stand. Without tensing the muscles of your legs, buttocks or belly, imagine that you're trying to hold back gas or a bowel movement. Try to isolate and tighten the ring of muscle around your vagina and your anus. Make sure you are not using the muscles of your abdomen or buttocks—put your hands on them, and if you feel movement, continue to experiment until you have isolated the pelvic floor muscles.

2. When urinating, empty your bladder partially, then try to stop or slow the flow of urine in midstream. The muscles that you use to do this are your pelvic floor muscles. Then relax and completely empty your bladder. Repeat this test twice a month to see if your pelvic floor muscles are getting stronger. With time it should get easier, and you will be able to contract these muscles for longer periods of time.

Step 2: Strengthen Those Muscles!

When you start these exercises, do the Kegels lying down to reduce stress on your muscles. Lie on your back and bend your knees or elevate your feet on a pillow. You should be comfortable and your legs should be relaxed, since tensing your other muscles or holding your breath will make it difficult for the pelvic floor muscles to work correctly.

Working from back to front, tighten your pelvic floor muscles and count to four slowly. Then release. The rest of your body should be completely relaxed. Do not tighten your abdominal, thigh or buttock muscles. Exhale as you contract, inhale as you release. Stop and rest when you are no longer performing each contraction properly.

As you get stronger, you can do these exercises anywhere—sitting or standing, while watching TV or waiting for a bus.

sitting in front of a computer. Breathing the right way will result in an increased oxygen intake that can buy you more energy, less stress, a clearer mind and better health in general.

There's more to deep breathing than simply filling your lungs with air. On the following pages you'll find eight breathing techniques that offer benefits ranging from a quick pick-me-up to lower blood pressure.

Health: Body Sense for Women

Try to do five to ten breathing exercises a day, either different ones or the same one, depending on how you're feeling.

Whenever possible, do them in a quiet, relaxed setting. If possible, turn off the phone ringer, shut down your computer and loosen your clothing.

(Caution: If you have heart disease, high blood pressure or have had a stroke, consult your doctor before trying a technique that involves holding your breath.)

The Basics

Abdominal Breathing. This is good for instant relaxation and also the starting point for several exercises that follow.

- Lie down on your back or sit comfortably.
- Place your hands on your abdomen.
- Inhale slowly and deeply, breathing air all the way down into the lower lobes of your lungs. As these fill with air, your lower belly should expand like a balloon. (Keep one hand on it so you can feel this happening.)
- Exhale slowly, allowing your abdomen to deflate as your body releases stale air.
- Inhale easily. Feel your belly expand again.
- Repeat for three to five minutes.

Yogic Breathing. This ancient technique promotes calmness and clarity of thought.

- Sit in a comfortable position (in a chair or cross-legged on the floor).
- Begin with one to two minutes of Abdominal Breathing.
- Close your right nostril with your right thumb and inhale through your left nostril for two counts.
- Close your left nostril with your right ring finger and hold your breath for eight counts. (Both nostrils are now closed.)
- Open your right nostril and exhale through it for four counts.
- Inhale through your open right nostril for two counts.
- Close your right nostril and hold your breath for eight counts.
- Open your left nostril and exhale through it for four counts.
- Repeat for 3 to 8 minutes.

Note: Your counts should be slow and consistent. If you feel fidgety, rock your body back and forth slowly.

Restorative Breathing

The Morning Revitalizer. Doing this exercise before you get out of bed each morning will help fill you with energy and make you more productive throughout the day. Follow it with some energizing stretches for the ultimate pick-me-up.

Note: Keep your eyes open throughout the exercise.
- Lie on your back in bed.
- Inhale through your nose as you raise your arms straight up toward the ceiling.
- Exhale through your mouth as you let your arms drop back onto the bed.
- Slowly repeat the last two steps six times.
- Exhale forcefully through your mouth while pulling your tummy in, then sit up.
- Inhale through your nose and reach your hands toward the ceiling.
- Exhale through your mouth as you pull your hands down to your shoulders and make tight fists.
- Repeat the last two steps four times.
- When you feel ready, swing your feet out of bed and move forward with enthusiasm and energy!

The Stress Buster. This technique helps you let go of anxiety and tension. Do it hourly, whenever you're at work or under a lot of pressure.
- Lie down on your back or sit up in a comfortable chair where you will not be disturbed.
- Relax with several Abdominal Breaths, breathing in for four counts, allowing your abdomen to balloon as the lower part of your lungs fills with air, then exhaling for eight counts.
- Take a deep breath through your nose and hold it as long as you comfortably can while tensing your feet.
- Relax your feet as you exhale through your mouth with a loud sigh: "AHHHHHHhhhhhhhh."
- Take a few Abdominal Breaths.
- Take a deep breath through your nose and hold it as you tense your calves.
- Relax your calves as you exhale through your mouth with a loud sigh: "AHHHHHHhhhhhhhh."
- Repeat for each area of the body, working from your feet up to your thighs, buttocks, abdomen, fingers, forearms, upper arms, shoulders and face.

Note: If you have limited time, mentally scan your body and focus your breath directly into the spots that feel tense. Try to move the affected area if possible—for example, shrug your shoulders or roll your neck.

Blood Pressure Reducer. Any relaxing type of breath can help control and reduce high blood pressure.

- Sitting comfortably in a quiet place, relax with a few Abdominal Breaths: four counts in, eight counts out.
- Inhale to about two-thirds lung capacity for about four counts. (Inhaling to only two-thirds of your maximum will help prevent an unintentional rise in blood pressure.)
- Hold for eight counts.
- Exhale for eight counts.
- Continue the two-thirds breaths for 3 to 8 minutes.

The Mood Booster. Try this breath whenever you're down in the dumps or feeling low-energy and blah.

- Stand with your arms at your sides, relaxed and with good posture.
- On a slow, steady inhalation, raise your arms horizontally until they're even with your shoulders.
- Move your arms in front of you. Finally raise your arms over your head.
- Exhale sharply through your mouth—make a "ha!" sound—while simultaneously dropping your head, neck and arms. Your body should be loose at the moment of exhalation.
- Repeat three to five times.

The Energizer. Beat the three o'clock doldrums with this uplifting trick.

- Do one to two minutes of Abdominal Breathing.
- Place your finger on your right nostril gently to help close its air flow.
- Take a deep, long breath in.
- Expel air through your left nostril, using short, forceful exhalations, as you pull in your abdominal muscles. Continue this staccato exhalation until your lungs are completely empty.
- Repeat 10 times.
- Do 1 minute of Abdominal Breaths.
- Inhale to about two-thirds of your lung capacity and hold it as long as comfortable before exhaling.
- Repeat the staccato breaths 10 times through your right nostril, placing your finger on your left nostril.
- Finish with one minute of Abdominal Breaths.

Ease the Pain. This breathing technique can help whether you have chronic back pain or you have merely stubbed your toe.

- Close your eyes and keep them closed throughout.

- Begin with an Abdominal Breath.
- Imagine pain leaving your body like a vapor or stream of color with each exhalation.
- Imagine your incoming breath traveling to the area of discomfort like a soothing balm.
- Release tension by wiggling various parts of your body as you breathe in and out.
- Release any emotion related to your pain by crying or sighing loudly. Don't keep this emotion bottled up. Let go of those painful feelings!
- Repeat for 4 to 8 minutes.
- As soon as you're ready, open your eyes. Stretch your arms and legs before getting up.

Calm Your Nerves. This instantly soothing exercise can minimize tension, whether you're stuck in line or fighting a traffic jam. Or try it right before bed and you'll sleep like a baby!

- Do deep Abdominal Breaths with long, slow exhalations.
- As you exhale, let go of any tension that you're holding in your body. Picture aggravation and worry drifting away with each exhalation.
- Imagine that with each inhalation you are filling your body with strength and the ability to solve problems.
- Realize that impatience will not get you to the head of the line faster. It will only make the time seem longer and increase your aggravation.
- Think of those around you as fellow human beings who are working to the best of their abilities.
- Continue breathing in and out as you imagine how great it would be if everyone else were relaxed and trying new ways to be patient and efficient.

YOUR 28-DAY CHALLENGE

Look at you! You've made your way through the health section, and you're more than halfway up the pyramid. Now I want you to think of your specific health goals. Do you need to make an appointment for a skin exam? Start doing deep breathing exercises every day? Go to bed earlier? Or put together a family health history to add to your health résumé? Pick four goals to work on for the next four weeks and write them down here.

Week 1: _____

_____

_____

_____

Week 2: _____

_____

_____

_____

Week 3: _____

_____

_____

_____

Week 4: _____

_____

_____

_____

If you've mastered all your goals at the end of four weeks, give yourself a healthy reward: Buy a great bottle of bubble bath, send in a subscription to a health magazine or rent your favorite funny movie.

6

Beauty: Erase the Signs of Aging

We've all heard the saying that beauty is only skin deep—and most of us know that this familiar phrase is true in more ways than one. Your skin is the largest organ in your body, and while we may not be accustomed to thinking about how our insides—our heart, arteries, bones, and muscles—are aging, we're usually very aware of the outward signs.

In your 20s you didn't give a whole lot of thought to your skin care routine. You ate whatever you wanted, spent hours in the sun, stayed up all night, even slept with makeup on. No problem! But now that time has started to catch up with you, you may be noticing some signs of neglect on your face. You've got dark circles that just won't go away and funny brown spots and blotches on your cheeks and forehead. Your skin seems to be flaky and always dry. You see deep lines around your eyes and mouth. And they all seemed to appear overnight.

You can't change the past, but there are some simple steps you can take to prevent future damage. And if you're willing to put in a little effort, you can actually erase some of those dark spots, lines and wrinkles. The key is to start now—before the problems get worse.

Believe me, I don't like to spend any more time getting ready in the morning than you do. A complicated beauty routine just isn't realistic—especially with a full-time job and two kids! So I've simplified the process by creating the easy-to-remember Seven-S Skin Saver Steps. If you can remember the letter S, you're on your way to younger-looking skin.

For those of you who have a little more time on your hands, I've included recipes for homemade oatmeal masks, the perfect pampering bath, treats for your tired eyes and secrets for creating your very own home spa—and trust me, these little extras are worth it. I've also included my Facial Fidgetcizers to help firm up those chin muscles and keep your face looking smooth and taut. My dear friend Jack LaLanne (yes, that fitness guru you've seen on TV for decades) swears by exercises like these. Take one look at his 85-year-old face and you'll know they work! And you don't need any extra time—you can do chin lifts while sitting at your desk, on a train or in your car, standing in line at the supermarket or watching TV. The trick is remembering to do them. But don't worry—I'll help you with that, too.

Throughout this section I'll also explain how the foods we eat and the activities we participate in all directly affect how we look and age. We've all met the older woman who glows like a 30-something or the elderly gentleman with movie-star good looks. Ask his or her secret, and you often get similar responses: exercising and eating right.

Can it be that simple? Yes. Feeling good comes from healthful choices, exercise and nutritional foods. And looking good comes from feeling good and using the tips that you're about to learn. So let's get started with the first things that we want other people to see—beautiful skin and a gorgeous smile. Here are my secrets for making sure your face shimmers with a youthful glow and radiance.

SKIN ESSENTIALS: SEVEN-S SKIN SAVER STEPS

Next time you see a baby, take a good long look at that newborn skin. It's clear, soft, flawless and full of natural color. Now look closely at the skin of the next woman you see. A quick comparison shows you the little lines and spots that come from our environment and our bad habits—too much sun, too little sleep, too much stress and too little exercise, to name a few. Following my Seven-S steps will help you focus on the ingredients to healthy skin—and help you achieve it!

1. **Stop smoking.** What's true for your heart is also true for your skin—smoking is bad! Smoking reduces the supply of oxygen in your blood and replaces it with carbon monoxide, which causes blood vessels to narrow. This decreases the flow of oxygen to your continually growing skin cells. The end result: premature wrinkling, especially around the mouth. Just take a look at a longtime smoker and you'll see what I mean! If you smoke, quitting today is the best thing you can do for yourself—both inside and out.

2. Wear sunblock. Ninety percent of sun damage and the wrinkles that result can be prevented with sunscreen, protective clothing (a hat, long pants and long sleeves) and sunglasses (to shield your eyes as well as the surrounding skin). Use a regular moisturizer with SPF 15 or higher (even on cloudy days)—that way you won't forget the sunscreen. Many cosmetic companies offer gentle, nongreasy moisturizers with sunblock that won't cause skin breakouts. If you spend a lot of time outside, don't forget to reapply it. You'll get all that bone-building vitamin D from the sun without the sunburn that can lead to skin damage. An ounce of prevention now will bring big results 10, 15, 20 years from now. Of course, the smartest thing to do to prevent sun damage is to limit your direct exposure as much as possible by covering up and sticking to shaded areas. But since this isn't always possible, try to be sun smart.

Sun Alternative: A Beautiful Golden Glow from a Bottle

Let's face it. The only healthy tan comes from a tube.

There are hundreds of self-tanners on the market now, but finding the right one isn't easy. This is the one area where spending a little more money is worth it. Inexpensive self-tanners often leave you looking orange or unnatural. So take a trip to the cosmetic counter. (Estée Lauder has a number of popular Go Bronze ones. Do some testing.) I like Bobbi Brown self-tanning gel for the face, and I prefer Clarins Self Tanning Milk for my legs and arms because it also has a sunscreen. If you don't want a full-blown tan but simply want to add a little color to your cheeks, mix a few drops of a cream-based tanner with a few drops of your favorite moisturizer and apply to your face each morning.

3. Slather on the moisturizer. With so many factors stealing moisture from our skin, we need to find a way to rehydrate. Store shelves and cosmetic counters are loaded with different moisturizers. So what works? A lot depends on where you live, the time of year and your individual skin type. During the winter months, especially in cold climates, a heavy cream is your best bet. When the temperatures rise, switch to a lighter moisturizing lotion. Try to find a product containing sunscreen—it's one less thing for you to worry about! Use the testers and find a product that works for you. Concentrate on the feel, ingredients, fragrance and benefits. And remember, expensive doesn't mean better.

If you're going to be out all day, bring along a purse-size moisturizer for quick re-applications.

4. Sip, sip, sip your water. You know all that water you've been drinking? I bet you're starting to notice a new softness and clarity to your complexion.

Moisturizing Makeover

As we age we need to apply moisturizer to places we often overlook. Many consider these areas of the body to be the true "age indicators." So, as you slather on your lotion, don't forget these spots:

Elbows
Hands
Knees
Heels
Feet
Neck
Earlobes
Eyebrows

Hydration Tip

For every hour you fly, drink at least one 8-ounce glass of water—not coffee or soda—to fight jet lag and keep your skin from drying out.

Water moisturizes your body from within and helps maintain the natural oils in the skin. It also helps the body to pump a healthy flow of nutrients from head to toe. Constantly sipping H_2O is one of the best things that I do for my complexion. Knowing that you'll see the benefits in the mirror should make drinking your 8 to 10 daily glasses a little easier!

Water Rescue

Here are my tips for making your H_2O a pleasure—not a punishment!

Citrus squeeze: Take a wedge of your favorite citrus fruit—lemon, lime, orange or grapefruit—and squeeze it into a glass of water. It adds a burst of flavor to tap water!

Cucumber water: Cucumbers aren't just for salad! Cucumbers are cooling and subtle, adding a wonderful taste to your water. Simply wash and peel a cucumber and add a few slices to your glass. For even more flavor, fill a pitcher with water, add four or five slices of cucumber, and allow to sit in the refrigerator for an hour or so.

Try bottled: If your local water simply doesn't taste good, bottled water may change your mind about swallowing a quick 8 ounces. (Or think about investing in a water purifier.)

Super splash: Add a splash of any juice (cranberry, grapefruit, lime or tangerine, for example) to your water glass. You'll love the flavor and the extra vitamin C.

5. Sleep. Sleep not only makes us feel wonderful, it is a beauty essential. Our bodies rejuvenate and repair themselves while we sleep. The telltale signs of too little sleep—dark circles and puffy eyes—are really an indication that we didn't give our bodies a chance to repair the damage of the previous day. A good eight hours also reduces stress and anxiety, and we all know that we don't look our best when we're stressed out. So get your sleep—it's a powerful beauty aid!

6. Step lively. In other words, EXERCISE! Look in the mirror the next time you finish exercising. The face looking back will be glowing—flushed with energy and radiance. Why? When we exercise, we pump blood throughout our bodies. Oxygen is delivered to every cell and organ, including our skin. We feel great, and we look even greater. Who needs a better incentive to move, move, move? Don't believe me? Take a brisk 10-minute walk before your next party or dinner date. It will be less than 10 minutes before you hear how great you look. When you take care of yourself, it shows!

Re-eye-tilize

Here are my tricks for getting rid of those dark circles and puffy eyes (no matter why you have them):

Cucumber quickie: Lie down with a slice of fresh cucumber over each of your closed eyes. The coolness of the cucumber soothes tired eyes while providing much-needed moisture. Your baby blues or browns will be rejuvenated and refreshed. This is wonderful if you've spent the day in front of a computer.

Tea bag trick: Steep two herbal tea bags and allow them to sit until slightly warm. Apply under-eye moisturizer around your eyes. Place the tea bags over your eyes and lie still for five minutes. The tea bags act as a soothing agent to relax stressed and puffy eyes. Next thing you know, the puffiness will be gone. Be sure to use herbal tea bags—the tannin in regular tea bags may stain your skin.

Cool it: Run a washcloth under cold water until saturated, then wring it out. Fold the cloth and rest it on your eyes for five minutes. Or try a commercial eye mask that you keep in the freezer for a quick eye treat. The cooling reduces both dark circles and puffiness. It's one of my favorite refreshers before an evening out.

7. **Stay sober.** While light alcohol consumption (one drink a day) won't damage your skin, excessive drinking dehydrates the skin, taking away what natural moisture it has. It also stimulates blood vessels, contributing to a condition called rosacea that's characterized by red, bumpy skin. Excessive drinking is also more likely to result in poor eating choices and a lack of exercise. And let's not forget bloodshot eyes—not a good look at any age!

Won't Working Out Make It Harder to Fall Asleep?

Some people say that a P.M. workout makes for a sound night's sleep, while others say that it keeps them awake. If you find that exercise is affecting your ZZZs, try working out in the morning or during the day. If time is an issue, break your exercise routine up into 10-minute segments and spread them throughout your day. Or if you're just not a morning person and mid-day workouts are impossible, do your workout as soon as you get home from work, so you have enough time to unwind before bed. Personally, I like to do my more rigorous workouts in the morning and a little relaxing activity in the evening: a stroll, yoga or stretching. Like all exercise programs, find what works for you!

THE ESSENTIAL AGE-DEFYING EXTRAS

My Seven-S Skin Saver Steps will help keep that old clock from springing ahead . . . but actually turning back the hands requires a little extra effort. Here are my Essential Extras for younger, more beautiful-looking skin (you'll find my home spa recipes on pages 258 to 259):

Exfoliate. When we're young, we generate new skin cells every two to three weeks. As we age, the process takes longer—up to six weeks in our 70s and 80s. When new cell growth slows down, we are left with older, flatter-looking and duller skin for an extended period of time. What can we do? We can help shed the dead skin cells and jump-start the regeneration process through gentle exfoliation. It's a natural way to give your skin a lift and keep you looking younger. There are many exfoliating products on the market—scrubs, grainy soaps, clay masks and others. The product that's right for you depends on your skin type, so seek some professional advice before making a selection. I use two different products—a stronger, grainy exfoliant once a week and a light scrub two to three times a week. Too much exfoliation can cause redness and irritation, so be careful not to overdo it.

Give yourself a facial. I try to get a professional facial every six weeks. Facials deep-clean your pores, remove dead skin cells and increase your blood circulation, bringing vital nutrients to the skin's surface. Fortu-

Don't forget your neck! Whatever you do for your face, do for your neck. The skin on your neck is similarly fragile and requires the same Seven-S Skin Saver Steps and Essential Extras.

Exfoliating Dos and Don'ts

Don't rush. If you are using an exfoliating mask, allow it to stay on your face for the recommended period of time. Rushing the process will decrease the benefits.

Do use your hands. Exfoliating aids like loofahs and mitts can be very damaging to sensitive facial skin. So use your hands—they are the best tools you have for exfoliating your skin.

Don't rough it. Your skin is sensitive, so you need to be gentle. Don't take out the day's aggressions on your skin by rubbing too hard. Also, look for a product that contains mild abrasives rather than extremely harsh particles. It's important to test the product before you buy it. Focus on the texture and feel of the product.

Do moisturize. When you have completed the exfoliating process, apply a light moisturizer to your damp skin. It will be absorbed quickly, leaving your skin soft and refreshed.

Exfoliate from Head to Toe!

Not only will your face benefit from exfoliating, you entire body (don't forget your feet) will rejoice when you remove those flaky dead skin cells. Almost every cosmetic line today includes terrific body scrubs and—my favorite—sea salt exfoliants. Once a week, take the time for a quick body sloughing when you're in the shower. You will notice a difference immediately. But be careful: Depending on the ingredients, some exfoliants can sting if you have a small cut or have recently shaved your legs.

nately, you don't have to go to a ritzy day spa or spend a lot of money to take advantage of this Essential Extra. About twice a week I do an at-home facial that includes a moisturizing mask, either in the morning before working out or right before bed. You'll find great recipes on page 258.

Get steamed. One of the best ways to really cleanse your skin is a simple steaming. Steaming relaxes your facial muscles, increases circulation and removes dirt and makeup from your pores. It also helps to loosen some of the dead skin cells to prepare your face for exfoliation. While it's tempting to simply hold your head over the pot of boiling pasta, creating an aromatic steam is better for your skin (and your soul). Fill a large bowl with some of your favorite herbs (I use peppermint, lavender and rosemary) and cover with boiling water. Place your face over the bowl and cover your head and the bowl with a towel. Steam your face for about five minutes. Follow it up with a splash of warm water and your favorite moisturizer. Don't you feel wonderful?

Fight the spots. For many women, the first visible signs of aging appear in the form of brown spots on our hands. What can we do to erase those icky age spots? Try this quick trick: Grate four radishes. Slowly add just enough plain yogurt to create a paste. Apply to the offending spot and leave on for about 10 minutes. Try this every other day until this natural bleach starts to work its magic.

Try a wrinkle-fighter. Retinol and alpha hydroxy acids (AHAs) can be found in a variety of products at the drugstore as well as department stores and spas. AHAs—glycolic or fruit acids added to many moisturizers and facial cleansers—help make your skin look and feel younger by promoting the growth of new cells (it's another, speedier method of exfoliation). And maybe you've heard of the prescription drug Retin-A and its wondrous effects. Now you can get a milder, over-the-counter version of retinoic acid (a form of vitamin A) called Retinol. The effects of Retinol are subtle and especially good if you have sensitive skin. Regular use of a product with Retinol can help repair sun-damaged skin, reduce the appearance of wrinkles and even out skin color. Retinol can be found in many products, from facial moisturizers to hand cream (it's great for those age spots!). It may take a few tries to find the right product for you—but it's worth it.

Stop picking. We all get blemishes for a variety of reasons. And when we do, the first inclination is to remove the villain. But before you act, remember that picking a blemish often results in bleeding and a scab (and maybe a scar), with a longer healing time. So instead, take action another way. Apply a topical blemish fighter and coverup. It's not the same as clear skin, but in the long run the result will be better. Or try applying an ice cube to the spot for several minutes—an insider tip from my favorite facialist!

Lip service. While we may take the time to throw on a little lipstick, we often forget about really taking care of our kissers. Just like your skin, your lips need protection from the sun. Try zinc oxide (sunscreen for your lips) or one of the many lipsticks available today with SPF. Your lips need moisture, too—try a petrolatum based lip cream or balm to protect your lips from the elements, especially if you spend a lot of time outside like I do. When lips are chapped, apply a balm immediately to prevent further drying and cracking.

Instant Makeovers

Need a quick fix to make you look your best? Here are my favorite quickies for looking your best:

Add some color. Nothing says youth and health like rosy cheeks. So stand up and do 10 quick jumping jacks or jog in place for 60 seconds. A quick burst of activity gives you a natural glow that no blush ever will.

Smile. A smiling face is the most beautiful face in the world. You'll look great and you'll feel great. So smile!

Eye energizer. Super fast and super easy! Grab an ice cube and lightly pat it on your eyelids and under your eyes. Your eyes are instantly awakened and energized!

Perfect posture. Stand up straight! When you do, you look strong, thin, confident and beautiful. If you don't believe me, look at yourself in a storefront window the next time you are walking down the street. Then stand up straight. The change is amazing!

Bar Exam: Does It Matter What Soap You Use?

Traditional bar soap (including many facial bar soaps) is extremely drying, robbing skin of natural oils and moisture. Most liquid soaps are also filled with moisture grabbers. Too much washing can also sap your skin of moisture. So look for a cleanser that is pH-balanced and has added moisturizers.

Face cleansing. If you have normal to oily skin, try a foaming cleanser. If you are oily all over, try a gel cleanser or oil-free cleansing product. If you have dry or sensitive skin, which many of us develop as we age, try a cleansing milk, cold cream or cleansing lotion. My suggestion: Read the labels and find a cleanser that is designed for your skin type, but pass by the bars—at least when it comes to your face.

Body bath. Traditional bar soaps can dry out the skin on the rest of your body as well. I try to pick a moisturizing bar, such as Dove or Oil of Olay. The liquid body washes found in most drugstores and supermarkets provide another less-drying alternative. Some even offer great scents for an A.M. pick-me-up or evening cool-down. Have fun experimenting with sample sizes until you find the product that works best for you.

Antibacterial options. While the thought of killing all those nasty germs sounds great, think again. Antibacterial soaps and cleansers are harsh and extremely drying—especially to facial skin. And lately experts have been warning that use of these antibacterial products may cause new strains of super-resistant bugs to emerge. Soaping up with a good moisturizing bar or a little liquid wash is enough to rid yourself of microscopic enemies. So skip the germ killers and save your skin instead.

SUPER LOCKS

Like your skin, your hair speaks volumes about your health and your age. A little extra attention to your mane will help you feel and look younger. Using a gentle shampoo and a good conditioner will help combat the dryness that develops with age. Try not to wash your hair every day. Water dries out your hair, causing it to break and become damaged. Use warm or cool water instead of hot, which is extremely drying for both your hair and your skin. Too many hair products also rob your hair of moisture. So take a weekend off from drying styling gels and mousses (especially products containing alcohol). Your locks will love you for it!

When you step out of the shower, gently towel-dry your hair. Working your locks too severely with a towel can result in hair loss or broken strands. Whenever possible, try to let your hair dry naturally. Constant use of hair dryers, curling irons and rollers will cause dryness and damage.

As your body's ratio of female hormones to male hormones shifts in your 50s and 60s, your hair may begin to get thinner. Don't worry—there are many products available to add thickness to your tresses. Try styling volumizers that do not contain alcohol (for example, Aussie Leave-In Volumizer and Herbal Essences Natural Volume Root Volumizer) or shampoos for thinning or fine hair. It also helps to bend over and blow your hair dry from underneath. The volume this creates is amazing (although it makes Fidgetcize during your bathroom routine a challenge!). Another great treat for your hair is hot oil. If you have time, it's worth it to get the treatment at your local salon or at home. You may also want to talk to your stylist about a new cut to minimize the appearance of thinning hair. A great new haircut can work wonders!

Find the products that work with your hair type and color. (And remember, expensive doesn't necessarily mean better.)

A word about stress and hair loss: Do you remember reading about Princess Caroline of Monaco's hair loss in 1995 after her breakup with a boyfriend? There were painful pictures of her wearing scarves. It seems that there is a medical condition called post-traumatic hair stress disorder. Doctors now know that psychological trauma can cause hair to stop growing. If your hair loss is related to stress, it will most likely grow back within a few months. In the meantime, it's not a bad idea to ask your doctor for advice and to switch to a body-building shampoo and conditioner.

NAIL DOWN YOUR BEAUTY ROUTINE

Your hands and your nails give quick insight as to how many candles will be on your next birthday cake. Here are a few things you can do to look younger—hands down!

- Rub hydrogen peroxide on dull, yellow nails for an instant brightener. Top with clear topcoat for an instant manicure.
- Moisturize your cuticles.
- Don't pick, pull or cut your cuticles. Instead, push them back with a cuticle stick (available at any drugstore).
- Wear rubber gloves when doing dishes or housework—it will help you avoid the drying effects of detergents and hot water.
- Don't use your nails as a staple remover, letter opener or other household tool.
- Limit your use of nail polish removers.
- Avoid quick-dry polishes, which are extremely drying.

Don't stop with your nails! Spend some time on your hands and feet. Use a pumice stone on your feet to reduce calluses. Or try a relaxing foot bath and foot scrub to remove dead skin cells on your feet. Manicures and pedicures keep your digits looking terrific. Moisturizing your hands and feet is equally important, especially since our heels and hands can really show our age.

BEAUTY COMES FROM WITHIN

When we hear the expression "beauty comes from within," we often think that beauty is part of one's soul, one's being. While that's certainly true, beauty also comes from what is *in* us. And this you, and you alone, control.

As you learned in Chapter 4, the foods you eat directly affect your weight, your workouts and your emotions. They also affect your hair, nails and your skin. Like any other part of your body, your skin needs to be nourished and protected. Similarly, your hair and nails need a steady

---

Regain the Glow!

You're falling in love, expecting a tax refund, or getting a big promotion at work—and you're "glowing." A rosy complexion and shiny hair are symbols of happiness *and* health. While you can't always control the happiness in your life, you can create the healthy glow! Here are a few tricks to create that blissfully-in-love look every day.

Change your makeup. Changing your makeup routine can do wonders for your look and your mood. Many cosmetic counters offer free makeovers, so give it a try. Remember, you only have to buy a product if you want to. Don't wear makeup? Try a colored lip balm for a little change.

Highlight your hair or try a new cut. Nothing says wow like a new look. If you're really daring, experiment with a whole new color!

Massage your skin. A quick facial massage will add color and a healthy glow to your cheeks.

Take a catnap. A quick 40 winks—or a power nap, as I like to call it—is invigorating. You'll wake up refreshed and ready to take on your next challenge!

Break a sweat. Want some quick color? Get moving. A little exercise goes a long way to giving you a natural, healthful glow. If you need proof, walk around the block, then look in the mirror. You'll see a glow that you'll never get from a bottle.

supply of nutrients to maintain their luster. As we grow older and years of sun damage and poor eating habits take their toll on our bodies, good nutrition is more important than ever.

Our face is the first part of ourselves that we present to others. A radiant glow tells the world that you are happy, healthy and full of life. Likewise, thick, shiny locks and strong, gorgeous nails can make you look and feel years younger. Achieving that look is easy if you understand what specific nutrients contribute to cover girl beauty. We've already talked about water. Here are a few of the other age-defying secrets.

- **Vitamin A (beta-carotene):** This antioxidant helps protect against skin cancer and premature aging. It also helps prevent hair loss and keeps skin from becoming dry and scaly.
- **Vitamins B_6 and B_{12}:** A deficiency in B vitamins may result in lackluster hair and pale, dry, itchy skin.

Pampering Pleasures

Feeling pretty is often the first step to looking pretty.

Paint your toes. Although no one else may see your toes, there is nothing more fun than adding some energizing color to your feet. My favorite color for toes is hot pink, especially during the summer.

Buy a scented soap or moisturizer. When I really want to splurge, I pick up fragrant body washes or moisturizers. My current favorite is Origins Gloomaway. The grapefruit scent makes me feel like I'm sitting in a Florida citrus grove. You can also buy yummy scented soaps and lotions in the drugstore for a fraction of the price in department stores.

Get a new lightbulb. Replacing your standard 60-watt bulb in the bathroom with a pink one will soften the light, so those little imperfections are less noticeable. Okay, you may be fooling yourself, but it's important to feel good when you look in the mirror!

Wear something feminine. Add a bright scarf to your business pantsuit. Or try some sexy lingerie under your uniform. Only you may know it's there—but the feel of soft satin is your own personal reminder of how gorgeous you are.

Treat yourself to candlelight. Even if you're eating alone, light a candle at dinner. The soft, low light is relaxing and calming, especially after a busy day. Better yet, instead of turning on the TV, try reading at night with a few aromatherapy candles. The fragrance and mood you create will allow you to feel lovely, inside and out.

- **Vitamin C:** This super-antioxidant helps stop free radicals from damaging our skin. It's essential for skin elasticity, preventing dry hair and skin and promoting the flow of blood and oxygen to your skin. If applied topically, studies show, it may help prevent wrinkles and liver spots.
- **Vitamin E:** Another powerful antioxidant that helps prevent free-radical damage. As with vitamin C, topical use may protect the skin.
- **Selenium:** This antioxidant, present in seafood and nuts, may help protect against skin cancer.
- **Protein:** One daily serving of protein, especially from fish sources such as salmon, sardines and tuna, will promote healthy hair and nail growth as well as help regulate skin moisture and pigment.
- **Fat (unsaturated):** Essential fatty acids found in vegetable oils and foods like nuts and seeds are crucial for maintaining smooth, moist skin.

Sometimes what we don't eat is as important as what we do eat. Not only are some foods bad for your health, they also show up on the outside. Fatty, greasy foods offer no nutrition and may result in breakouts. Chocolate and hard cheeses are considered by many to be blemish makers. Let's not forget sugar-filled sodas. Don't believe me? Look in the mirror the day after a junk-food binge. You'll see the difference. So before you dive into a decadent dessert, take a peek in your powder compact. What more incentive do you need to order fresh berries?

Check pages 136 to 141 of the nutrition section for more details on what nutrients are good for your skin—and what foods you can find them in. Overall, healthy and balanced nutrition is the key. If you eat right and take supplements, beautiful, radiant skin will follow!

CREATE YOUR OWN HOME SPA

Many of my Lifetime shows are filmed at the country's most beautiful fitness resorts and spas. Between shoots I sometimes reward myself with a spa treatment. I especially love facials, pedicures and massages.

But as much as I love visiting these pampering palaces, the majority of my days are spent at home or in less luxurious locations. So I've learned to create my own home spa. Most of my home treatments can be made with ingredients that you probably already have in the pantry. You can take a whole day and indulge in several treatments, or do them one at a time as your schedule permits.

The best way to begin is by creating a spa atmosphere. Turn off the phone and the TV and turn on some soothing music. There are lots of

The Perfect Bath

1. Reserve 20 minutes.

2. Unplug the phone or turn off the ringer.

3. Place votive or aromatherapy candles along the edge of your bathtub or around your bathroom.

4. Pour coarse sea salts (¼ cup) or a combination of aromatherapy essential oils (I like to use a couple of drops of rosemary and lavender) into your bath. In a pinch, use two herbal tea bags. This is a wonderful way to encourage a good night's sleep.

5. Turn on some soft, soothing music.

6. Turn down the lights.

7. Relax and enjoy!

options out there—from classical to Celtic to New Age—that can help relax you. Dim the lights and set the mood with aromatherapy candles. Bright lights are very glaring and often keep you from unwinding. Take a few minutes to appreciate your spa surroundings. Now take a deep breath and enjoy whatever treatment you're indulging in!

Oatmeal Face Mask

Combine 2 tablespoons honey, ½ cup ground oatmeal and ¼ cup plain yogurt. Apply liberally to your face and neck (avoiding the eye area). Leave on for 15 minutes, then rinse with warm water.

Banana Face Mask

This is a great way to use up those overripe bananas! Mash 1 banana and add 1 tablespoon plain yogurt, 1 teaspoon honey and 1 tablespoon heavy cream. Apply this rich, creamy mask and wait 5 to 10 minutes before rinsing off.

Herbal Steams

Add the following herbs to boiling water for a refreshing steam:

Normal skin: Lavender, rosemary, chamomile and peppermint
Oily skin: Rosemary, sage, peppermint and basil
Dry skin: Lavender, rose, parsley and chamomile

Dry Skin Saver

Combine 1 tablespoon honey, 4 tablespoons olive oil and the juice of 1 lemon. Apply to all those dry, rough spots—your elbows, your heels and your knees—and massage for three minutes.

Sea Salt Exfoliater

Take 2 tablespoons of coarse sea salts (you can find them in most gourmet food stores) and add 2 tablespoons lemon juice. Step into the shower (without the water running) and moisturize your body with ½ cup olive oil. Then massage the salt mixture all over your skin for 10 minutes. When you're finished, rinse with warm water. You'll notice an instant difference!

Warm-Oil Hair Treatment

Heat ¼ to ½ cup of extra-virgin olive oil, depending on the length of your hair. While the oil is heating, take two towels (not your best ones) and toss them in the dryer to warm them up. When the oil is warm, massage it into your scalp and hair. Don't miss a single strand! When you are finished massaging, take one of the warm towels and create a turban around your head. Relax for 15 to 30 minutes. If the towel gets too cold, replace it with another warm towel. When you're ready, use a gentle shampoo to remove the oil from your hair.

Hot-Oil Nail Treatment

Heat ¼ cup of olive oil until warm to the touch. Add the vitamin E from one capsule and stir. Now massage the oil mixture into the cuticles on your hands and feet. If you have any left, massage it into your hands. If you do this regularly, you will notice a big change in the appearance of your nails.

YOUR 5-MINUTE NATURAL FACE-LIFT

The muscles of your face are no different from the muscles of your body: Proper exercise can build, tone and firm them. When the muscles aren't used, tissue begins to break down, becoming soft and loose. Facial exercises can help build up the muscles in and around your upper eye area, your cheekbones and your chin to restore a more youthful look. It's like training your facial muscles to minimize wrinkles and

Beauty: Erase the Signs of Aging

regain the natural contours of your face. Better blood flow adds up to better elasticity and cell renewal. You'll also help stimulate circulation to bring nutrients to the skin's surface. Imagine—just a few short minutes can lead to healthier-looking skin, no matter what your age.

There is real science behind this. When you're happy, report dermatologists, the blood flow to your skin increases, giving you a healthy flush. Your muscles relax, making your skin look smoother. The opposite is also true. When you're tense, your blood vessels and muscles constrict, causing sallow skin and, over time, a permanently furrowed brow.

I've created an easy 5-minute face routine that can be done at any time, anywhere—whatever works with your schedule. I like to do it at night after I've washed my face and put on a good moisturizer. This is a natural face-lift—no surgery required! It's safe, free, fast and a fabulous way to minimize a double chin. (Of course, don't forget about watching your diet and exercising your body, which is essential to getting rid of that extra fat.) Don't expect results overnight—but if you stick with Facial Fidgetcize, you can tighten the muscles of your face and neck to turn back your beauty clock.

In the next five minutes you're going to do three different things to give your face a lift: (1) a mini-massage to stimulate circulation, relax your muscles and increase blood flow; (2) Facial Fidgetcize—facial exercises to tone and lift and to reduce the appearance of wrinkles; and (3) acupressure to relax and release facial tension. Facial exercise is a gradual process, so do whatever's comfortable for you. Not only do I want you to look great, I want you to feel great.

Step 1: Massage

Your mini-massage begins with soothing, gentle strokes all over your face. This is wonderful if you've been thinking hard or squinting in front of a computer screen. Since you'll be touching your face, make sure your hands are clean. First, apply a light moisturizer to hydrate your skin. Next, cover your face with your hands and apply gentle pressure for 10 seconds. Move your fingertips to your forehead and lightly massage your temples, moving from your eyebrows up to your hairline. When you are finished, move your fingertips down so that they are located in the middle of your face (between your eyes and your mouth) and continue massaging with upward strokes. Eventually move your fingertips to your chin and neck and continue stroking. Ahhh, don't you feel relaxed? Now you're ready to do some Facial Fidgetcize!

Step 2: Facial Fidgetcize

Facial Fidgetcize is a terrific way to work and tone your facial muscles for an age-erasing workout. Like my other Fidgetcize exercises, Facial Fidgetcize is fast and flexible. You can do it in your car, in line at the store, in the ladies' room, at your desk. It's so simple, there's simply no reason NOT to do it!

Full Face Stretch. Sit or stand up straight. Open your eyes as wide as you can as you lift your eyebrows to the sky. Next, keeping your teeth covered with your lips, open your mouth as wide as you can. You'll feel a stretch from head to chin. Hold for 10 seconds.

Upper Eye Lift. Anchor your index fingers under your eyebrows, where the bone is. Your fingers will provide resistance. Using the muscles of your upper eyelid, press your eyebrow down against your fingers. This will strengthen your eye muscles, giving you the bright-eyed look of a 20-something. Hold for 10 seconds.

Cheekbone Toner. The goal of this exercise is to lift your cheekbone muscles, giving you greater definition. Begin by placing your index fingers beneath your eyes. Press down as you lift your cheeks up by smiling or forming an O with your mouth. Hold for 10 seconds.

Lion Pose. Borrowed from yoga, this exercise can help contour the lower part of your jawline, giving you a better side profile. You can do this in the car when you're waiting at a red light or when picking your kids up from school.
- Inhale deeply through your nose.
- Hold your breath for a few seconds while sticking out your tongue as far as possible (try to touch your chin). Open your eyes as wide as you can.
- Exhale through an open mouth, making an "ahhh" sound.

Neck Lift. Sitting up straight, move your lower lip up and over your upper lip. The stretch through your neck releases tension and works to give you an elegant Audrey Hepburn neck. Hold for five seconds.

Buy a Vowel. No, you're not on the game show *Wheel of Fortune*. Repeating the five vowels is actually an old-fashioned but very effective Facial Fidgetcizer. The idea is to exaggerate your enunciation of each letter to really use your facial muscles.

- Inhale deeply through your nose.
- Say the letter *A*. Open your mouth wide to the side in an exaggerated smile (or a Jim Carrey funny face) as you speak. Feel the stretch. Breathe in.
- Say the letter *E*. Exaggerate the sound by extending the lower jaw and moving your mouth. You'll feel a stretch under your chin. Breathe in.
- Say the letter *I*. Open your mouth as wide as you can as you say it. Breathe in.
- Say the letter *O*. Stretch your lips out in front of you as you bring them into an O shape. Breathe in.
- Say the letter *U*. Lower your chin. As you raise it say the letter *U*. You'll feel the lift and stretch in your neck.
- Repeat.

Step 3: Acupressure

Our bodies have many pressure points, especially on our heads. When we apply pressure directly to these spots, we release stress and tension. Acupressure is especially effective for headache and TMJ sufferers. Releasing tension will keep you from clenching your teeth and furrowing your brow—a real wrinkle creator! But don't press too hard, since you don't want to injure any blood vessels.

- Hold your ears and rotate them in a circular motion—forward five times, then backward five times. Next, press the skull bone behind your ears. We all hold a great deal of tension in this part of our body, so it's important to release this stress.
- Press right above the center of your eyebrows and gently press and pull as you work your way to the corners of your eyes. When you reach the outside of your eyebrows, gently pull your eyebrows toward your ears to release tension in your brow and smooth away wrinkles.
- Starting right below your earlobes, gently press all along your jawline as you move down toward your chin. Feel the stress of the day evaporate.
- Finish by covering your face with your hands and press slightly. For me, this is a wonderful way to end the day and to fall into a deep, peaceful sleep.

Before Bed: My Basic Beauty Routine

- Cleanse face to remove dirt and makeup (never sleep with makeup on!).

- Twice a week use a soft, slightly grainy scrub to slough off dead skin cells (once a week I use a stronger, grainier exfoliating scrub). I like Never a Dull Moment by Origins or my homemade oatmeal mask.

- Smooth on moisturizer. (I alternate between a Retinol cream that I get from my facialist and a vitamin C lotion from my local health food store.)

- Gently apply a light eye cream.

- Do a few minutes of Facial Fidgetcize!

- Rub hydrating lotion on my elbows, hands and feet. The newest lotion by Keri with AHAs is terrific.

- Use a lanolin-based gel with petrolatum on my lips.

- Climb into bed for a rejuvenating 8-hour slumber.

YOUR 28-DAY CHALLENGE

Now it's time to set your beauty goals for the next four weeks. Think about the areas that concern you most and use them as starting places. If you haven't been using sunscreen, drinking enough water, or getting enough shut-eye, these are excellent places to begin. Your actual goals might be to switch to a moisturizer with SPF 15, bring a big water bottle to work, or go to bed 30 minutes earlier every night. Other goals might be to use an exfoliating scrub once a week, apply moisturizer to those flaky elbows and heels after showering or paint your toenails a fun fire-engine red. Ready to make your list? Let's do it!

Week 1: _____

_____

_____

_____

Week 2: _____

_____

_____

_____

Week 3: _____

_____

_____

_____

Week 4: _____

_____

_____

_____

A FINAL WORD: COSMETIC SURGERY

So many women are turning to plastic surgery now to turn back the clock—liposuction, tummy tucks, laser resurfacing. Millions are spent every year on our quest to look forever young.

I'm not against it (especially if it helps boost your self-esteem), but I know it's not for me—yet. And cosmetic surgery has certainly come a long way since the old days of the too-taut face-lift, which left aging divas, socialites and movie stars with a permanent look of astonishment on their faces. But today women—and men—are turning to cosmetic surgery at a younger age. In fact, the number of patients 34 and younger has more than doubled in the last decade. The emphasis seems to have shifted from looking younger to looking perfect.

I know of women who have chemical peels, which use a variety of alpha hydroxy acids to slough off skin cells and erase facial lines, acne scars and pigmentation problems. The danger here is that if the chemical is too high in acid or left on the skin too long, it can permanently burn or discolor your face. Women are also submitting to injections of Botox (a derivative of the deadly botulism poison, which temporarily paralyzes muscles to smooth out lines) and collagen, which temporarily plumps up lips or cheeks. Maybe I'm overly cautious, but I'd worry about being injected with a foreign substance, for whatever reason. So I'm willing to face my 40s with the face I deserve.

If you want to explore cosmetic surgery, make sure your doctor is board certified. You can determine this by calling the American Society for Dermatologic Surgery at 800-441-2737 or the American Society of Plastic and Reconstructive Surgeons at 800-635-0635.

In addition, many facialists now specialize in nonsurgical face-lifts.

These unique treatments restore a natural, healthy glow with the help of electrical currents or acupressure. These facials are expensive (about $150–200 a session) but are a welcome alternative for women who are looking for safer, less invasive remedies. Ultimately, the choice is yours. Just remember: We all want to look and feel our best, but a perfect complexion is never a means to happiness.

A final word on beauty: Helena Rubenstein, the cosmetics queen who lived to be 95, said it best: "I have always felt that a woman has the right to treat the subject of her age with ambiguity until, perhaps, she passes into the realm of over ninety. Then it is better to be candid with herself and with the world."

7

Attitude: Stay Young at Heart!

Maybe you've dismissed the cliché "staying young at heart" as just that, a cliché. Well, it's time that your mind started listening to your heart again. Just look around. See that grandmother at your local playground? There she is on the swings or in the sandbox with the grandkids, looking happy and relaxed. And what about the older gentleman on the block who is always chuckling or cracking jokes? He may have a few laugh lines, but his cheeks are rosy and his eyes twinkle.

As you know, I'm a true believer in a positive, think-young attitude. It's a crucial part of my formula for creating happiness in every facet of your life. A positive outlook can help minimize the stress that leads to illness, prevent frown lines that make you look old and dour, and make you the type of person that others—old or young—enjoy spending time with.

My sisters, brother and I are all alike—we love to laugh at ourselves and each other. My grandmother was so funny; she was like a magnet, everyone just loved to be around her. But a youthful outlook doesn't come naturally for everyone. Just like good exercise, eating and health habits, it can require thought and effort. In this chapter I'll share with you my very own secrets for developing a healthy attitude and getting more out of life. You'll also learn how to eliminate the negative thoughts that may be preventing you from leading a full, active life or that may be sabotaging your efforts to trim down and stay in shape.

As the architects of our own lives, we all have the ability to shape our future. But this is often the first thing we lose sight of when we're overwhelmed by work and worries about money, our kids and "getting it all done." Think about athletes who choke in the big game. Why does it happen? Sports psychologists will tell you that it's because their minds aren't truly focused on the task at hand or they question their ability to win. The same goes for looking and feeling young—you need confidence and concentration to win the anti-aging game, too. If your mind and heart aren't fully invested, you'll have trouble getting the results you're after.

The mind-body connection is controlled by a master gland called the hypothalamus. This all-important connector is located near where your brain and spinal cord join. Together with your hypothalamus, a complex set of nerves and biochemicals sends messages back and forth between your brain and the rest of your body. The key is sending the *right* messages.

For 5,000 years yoga practitioners have preached the power of the mind to improve physical health. Scientific research also suggests the incredible impact that a positive attitude can have on your immune system. People with optimistic outlooks have fewer illnesses and recover from injuries and diseases more quickly. According to one study, optimists can live as much as 20 percent longer than pessimists. The choice could be yours: You can think yourself sick or think yourself well.

The power of positive thinking extends beyond your health. Picture a pregnant woman or a blushing bride. When you're happy, it shows on the outside. You smile a lot and your skin glows. You're more fun to be around. A positive outlook also makes it easier for you to get out there and exercise, eat right and take care of yourself. What better reason to think of your glass as half full?

I'm lucky: I was born a happy person. And I'm convinced that optimism has helped keep me young and healthy. It's also opened doors in my career. I didn't get to be a regular on *The Jack LaLanne Show* because I could do 50 sit-ups in a minute. Jack gave me my first big break because he knows that a positive attitude is an instrumental and essential element of physical fitness. The same is true for my first job as fitness correspondent for NBC's *Today* show. Anyone can teach an aerobics class, but the producers recognized that an upbeat personality will keep viewers motivated, excited, enthusiastic *and* tuned in. And I know my friend Don Imus would never invite me on his show unless I made him laugh!

Don't get me wrong—like you, I occasionally sweat the small stuff. But I snap out of it quickly because I know how much healthier it is and how much better it feels to approach life with a smile and to assume the best, not the worst.

Consider all the successful go-getters in the world—the Bill Gateses, Donald Trumps and Oprah Winfreys. Listen to them speak—they're

Attitude: Stay Young at Heart!

confident and optimistic. They talk about what they *can* do and what they *will* do. They aren't consumed with doubt and self-loathing. They use their positive attitudes to face challenges and overcome obstacles.

Sports and professional athletes are a big part of the Austin family's life. I've learned valuable lessons from these world-class winners—the most important being that you need to approach every game thinking, *and knowing*, that you can win. This GO, FIGHT, WIN attitude doesn't apply just to a bridge game or tennis match—it's how you should approach every single day.

How often do you hear yourself say, "I won't," or "I can't" or "I don't"? "I won't try tofu." "I can't lose weight." "I don't like to exercise." If you're like most people, you use negatives as a shield against new experiences. If you don't take risks, you'll have nothing to lose, right? Wrong! As the saying goes, the only things that you regret in life are the things that you don't do. So start right now by announcing to the world:

> I can.
> I will.
> I am.

Remember these words. Make them your new mantra. Repeat them to yourself several times a day. Believe that anything is possible!

As you embark on your anti-aging program, follow these 10 simple tips for staying young at heart:

1. SIMPLIFY YOUR LIFE

As employees, spouses and caretakers, it seems like there's always *something* demanding our time and attention. Practically every woman I know feels as though she has too much to do! When stress levels tend to soar and healthy habits often go out the window, who has time for a

---

Remember to compliment yourself. You don't like it when others criticize you, so don't criticize yourself.

Denise's Daily Dos

I have found these simple affirmations to be extremely effective in my own life. Give them a try!

1. It's a beautiful day—and I'm a beautiful part of it!

2. My family and friends love me.

3. I have 50 things on my to-do list, but I can and will get 5 things done today.

4. I'm going to smile at everyone today.

nutritious sit-down meal or eight hours of sleep? These may feel like small sacrifices at the time, but in the long run they'll take a toll on your health and well-being.

Stress is most often the result of time deficiency. Think about it: You're late for work or to pick up your kids, or you just have too much to do. You're edgy, tense and ready to snap at anyone or anything that gets in your way. Unfortunately, you can't quit your job, give up doing laundry or stop paying taxes. So what can you do to prevent those stress situations from happening? Here are a few of the things I do to keep tabs on my time and stay sane:

Get organized. An hour spent organizing your office or living quarters can save you a lot of frustration and make you more efficient and productive. Lists are another good way to stay on top of things. (Many women have found the new Palm Pilots indispensable.) At the start of each month I also sit down with my calendar to plot out the coming weeks. It doesn't take all day—only about 15 to 20 minutes.

Creating a Clutter-Free Calendar

Get a blank calendar and a box of colored markers and start working on creating a clutter-free four weeks. Begin by marking the must-dos on your calendar in red—doctor's appointments, exercise (yes, this is a not-so-subtle reminder) and important meetings and events. Next, plan out the incidentals for the month in blue: laundry, food shopping, car pools, dry cleaner and so on. In yellow, mark down the fun events in your week—taking a hike with friends, seeing the hottest flick or going shopping. Finally, use a green highlighter to mark off free time—at least a half hour each day. Using this color system will keep you from overloading any one day and will help you maintain a balanced schedule. And if it's not on your calendar, don't do it. Learning to organize is the first step to reducing the clutter in your life.

Set boundaries. Many of us pride ourselves on our productivity and time spent helping others. But you need to be realistic. Think about what you're actually able to do, and do well, in the time that you have. When you try to do too much, you often end up cutting corners, which can lead to aggravating mistakes. Instead, try limiting yourself to a few activities and do them well. For example, I'm often asked to do appearances for charities, both local and national. I can't be at every event, so I limit my participation to my three favorite charities. It's hard to say no, especially when you're used to saying yes. But your guilt won't last as long as the stress that comes from overextending yourself and not doing anything well.

Eliminate hidden "time eaters." Take a close look at your routine to determine where you may be wasting precious minutes. Do you make multiple trips to the grocery store during the week or spend a lot of time getting dressed in the morning? Learn to streamline your routine, and you'll find the spare time that you need to do things like exercise, eat right and get enough sleep.

Learn to delegate. Whether you're at home or in the office, don't be hesitant to ask for help. It isn't a sign of weakness. It's a smart way to free yourself up for more important tasks, such as exercising or providing balanced meals for your family. At home, I give my girls the job of setting the table (and have learned not to care if the spoons are in the wrong place). After dinner, Jeff pitches in by washing pots and putting the dishes in the dishwasher. He's happy to do it—by now, I don't even have to ask!

2. BELIEVE IN YOURSELF

If I didn't believe in myself, I wouldn't be where I am today. I didn't wake up one day and have my own national TV show. It was a long, arduous road, and I suffered a lot of rejection along the way. I can't even count the number of calls that I placed, letters that I sent, and ideas that I pitched. Twenty years ago, when I was just getting started, the aerobics and fitness industry was in its early stages, too. Many people thought that all that bouncing around was silly.

I finally made it into the national television circuit in the early 80s, when I landed a job as the first-ever fitness correspondent for the *Today* show. I had been trying to pitch the idea to the show's producer for weeks. I left message after message, but he didn't call me back. Finally I went to New York and staked him out one morning. As he approached his office building I ran up and handed him my promo tapes. I was terrified that he would think I was a stalker! But the persistence paid off: He watched the tape, and I was offered the dream job that really sent my career into orbit.

There are still plenty of times when I doubt myself. I have days when I look in the mirror and think, "Ugh!" or get nervous about getting up in front of a crowd of people to give a speech. Self-confidence isn't something that is automatic for most of us—so we have to work to continually build and reinforce it.

We all need to accept the fact that we're not perfect. Everyone has fat days, bad hair days, days when you change outfits a hundred times and still don't like what you see. It's just a part of life. You can't expect a complete attitude adjustment overnight. But you can start taking baby steps toward a better self-image. Perfectionism is a common problem with women over 40, and it can lead to feelings of depression. Remember, you're not perfect—you're just the perfect version of you!

The first step is to focus on your gifts. I truly believe that everyone is given a gift from God. My gift is the ability to make people happy. I've always been able to make others laugh. Growing up as a middle child, I was always the peacekeeper, the mediator. And in high school my classmates voted me "Most Friendly" and "Class Clown." Luckily for me, I've been able to make this gift work for me in my professional life, too.

What's your special gift? If you don't know, then try this simple exercise. Ask someone close to you to tell you what they like about you. Which of your qualities stand out as being special and unique? Write their comments down on an index card. Review the list every morning before getting out of bed and every night before going to sleep.

You are an incredible, unique individual with much to offer. So focus on what you *are* instead of what you *aren't*. Reprogram that little voice way down inside you with positives. Rather than say "fat" or "unattractive," think "smart, funny, interesting, motivated, giving, beautiful." Try to erase any memories of feeling like a failure or being embarrassed. Keep reminding yourself of your successes, no matter how small, and all that you give to your family and others.

Remember: People can sense your discontent whether you vocalize it or not. Your wide frown and droopy slouch send out signals that say, "I don't feel good about myself." So keep reminding yourself of your assets. And when you enter a room, do it with confidence: Hold your chin up, pull your shoulders back and smile—a big, wide smile! You are worthy—convince yourself, and others will believe it, too.

Right here, right now, I want you to write down five things that you *like* about yourself:

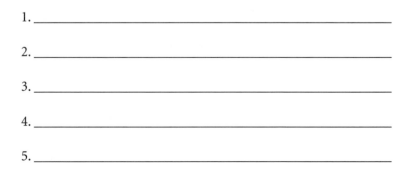

1. _____

2. _____

3. _____

4. _____

5. _____

Remind yourself of these attributes whenever you start feeling doubt or insecurity. Review your list of positives every night before you go to bed, or carry it with you so you can pull it out whenever those self-critical thoughts pop into your head. Don't let self-doubt become a self-fulfilling prophecy.

3. STAY CONNECTED WITH FRIENDS AND FAMILY

Nothing makes me feel happier than time spent with close friends and family members. It helps recharge my batteries and reminds me of what life is all about—love, companionship and simple pleasures.

Whether you're a 40-year-old mom or a housebound senior, it's important to have loved ones that you can count on for advice and who appreciate your opinions and efforts. This kind of positive support system is particularly crucial when you're making major lifestyle changes like starting an exercise program or trying to lose weight. Who better to share concerns about nagging personal problems with than your sister or a trusted friend?

A week after we were married, Jeff and I moved to Washington, D.C. He had been offered a great new job with a sports management firm. It was a great opportunity for him, so I encouraged the move, even though it meant leaving our families behind. For me, it also meant giving up my own early-morning TV show in Los Angeles. Our new home was terrific, but we didn't know anyone and I didn't have a job. After I was done unpacking and decorating, I got increasingly sad and depressed.

Fortunately, my parents and my siblings in California were just a phone call away. They really helped coach me through that tough time and countless others. I am so lucky to have a supportive family. Even though they live 3,000 miles away, I still see them about once a month and talk to one of them on the phone practically every day.

Seventeen years later Jeff and I have definitely settled in on the East Coast. We have a great group of friends whom we see regularly for dinner or a little tennis. About once every six months or so I also plan a special get-together with my best girlfriends—an afternoon of shopping, a hiking expedition or even a weekend getaway. Sometimes we include the kids, sometimes we don't.

Taking time to maintain or build healthy relationships isn't selfish— it's a vital part of the anti-aging equation. If you have young kids, get a

Ear Exercises

Here are a few practice tips for becoming a good listener:

1. **Count to 10 before you interrupt.** You'll think before you speak *and* give your friend a chance to finish her thought.

2. **Practice eye contact.** Nothing says "I'm listening" like eye contact. Practice on whomever you are talking to—your dry cleaner, your restaurant server, your boss or your significant other. The more comfortable you are with eye contact, the easier it becomes.

3. **Enact the 5-second drill.** Take a deep breath and wait for 5 seconds before responding to a question or comment. If you respond immediately, it looks as though you've been thinking about what you were going to say and not really listening.

4. **Concentrate.** When you really focus on what's being said, it shows. And there is nothing worse than having to ask a crying friend to repeat her breakup story because you were busy thinking about dinner or reading your E-mail.

baby-sitter or ask a neighbor to watch them while you go for a stroll with a friend. Call your sister or brother to catch up. Plan an evening with old college friends. In a pinch, use the phone or E-mail to stay in touch with family and friends. You'll feel reconnected and ready to take on the next challenge.

What if you just moved to a new neighborhood or city? Or maybe your family is small? Create a new network. Join a book group at your local library or bookstore. Take a continuing-education class at the local university. Volunteer at your synagogue or church. Start an investment club, picking out stocks and meeting for dinner once a month. The opportunities to connect are everywhere. It may take a little while to develop positive new friendships, but don't worry, it will happen.

Whom I spend my time with has become more and more important to me as I get older. Why waste all that precious time and energy on people who make you feel bad about yourself? While positive relationships can make life more interesting, exciting and fun, negative relationships do just the opposite. They suck the life out of you. Literally.

Take a moment right now to think about the people who surround you at work, at home and socially. Would you characterize them as optimists or pessimists? Do they make you feel good or sad? Relationships should be positive and invigorating forces in our lives. So if you're not getting the love and support you need, it's time to go out and find it.

4. REACH OUT TO OTHERS

What could be more spiritually uplifting than doing something nice for another person? Being altruistic doesn't have to mean donating your life savings to charity. You can give of yourself by asking a lonely widow in your neighborhood over for dinner or offering to baby-sit for a friend's kids. The best gifts in life are free—and they give back times three! Here are a few ways to reach out to those around you:

Volunteer. Spend a Saturday with your kids cleaning up a local park or lend a hand at your local soup kitchen. The community will benefit, and so will your muscles as you rake leaves or dish up dozens of meals. You'll realize how lucky you are and all that you have to offer. You'll feel appreciated and learn to revel in the joy of small gestures.

Help your children. Chaperone the high school dance. Become a Girl Scout leader. Be an assistant coach for your son's soccer team. Your children will see the importance of involvement, leadership and participation—and you'll gain inspiration to get off the couch along with priceless bonding opportunities. Don't have kids? No problem. Become a Big Sister or volunteer at the local school.

Be a good listener. Listening may be the ultimate example of selfless giving—and it's a gift that you can bestow every day. It can be tough to sit and listen to someone else's problems without jumping in and trying to solve them. Remember that the person doing the talking may not want advice—she simply may want to get her troubles off her chest. The best way to help may be to listen without offering your two cents.

Stress Rx

These are three of my favorite mini-therapies for stress:

Color therapy. There is nothing like a hot-pink dress, lime green blouse or red power suit to make you feel strong, and feeling strong and unshakable is a great first step in battling stress.

Music therapy. Listening to soothing music always helps me to unwind. Try a CD by Enya or a mellow New Age tape. Or if you're in the car, try singing away your stress. Belting out a favorite tune as loud as you can is instant therapy. (You'll just have to ignore the stares from other drivers!)

Walk it off. I often find that a quick burst of activity is the best way to shake off stress. If walking isn't an option, try the stairs or even a few jumping jacks.

5. ROLL WITH THE PUNCHES

As much as we'd like to, we can't control everything that happens to us. We'd all like to think that bad things won't happen, but they sometimes do. That's life. It isn't always fair. All you can do is brace yourself for the inevitable bumps in the road and try to get past them as smoothly and easily as possible.

Let's say you get into a car accident—and, thankfully, no one gets hurt. You have two options: You can berate the other driver for running a stop sign and causing the accident. Or you can use your cell phone to call 911 and start writing down the other driver's registration and insurance information. The damage is already done. Do you waste time and energy yelling, or do you try to make the best of it?

Whenever the road of life gets a little bumpy, picture yourself gliding over the potholes. Instead of pulling down the shades and hiding or freaking out, search for solutions. You have the power to solve almost any problem that comes your way. So don't waste energy sweating the small stuff—save it for more important tasks like working out or cheering your daughter on at her big softball game.

If you find yourself reacting to a stressful situation rather than rolling with it, do what I do—take a time-out. To calm yourself, try taking some deep breaths or doing some soothing stretches. Then imagine yourself floating in a beautiful, tropical blue sea or sitting on a mountain watching the sunset. Remember: An emotional breakdown won't help you out of a jam—all it will do is give you high blood pressure!

One of the best ways to prevent a major meltdown is by not letting stress build up in the first place. I'm more likely to let the pressure get to me when I feel bombarded by a million different things. Avoid letting it get to that level by maintaining balance in your life and practicing regular stress-reducing techniques like deep breathing and meditation.

Take a Deep Breath

We always hear people say to take a deep breath during stressful moments. But how exactly do you do this? Begin by standing or sitting up straight. Make sure your legs aren't crossed. If you can, close your eyes slightly. Focus your mind on the back of your throat and inhale slowly and deeply. Try to visualize your breath moving down your throat, into your lungs and further down into your belly. Hold for 3 seconds and slowly exhale. Reverse the visualization of the air leaving your belly, your lungs and then your mouth. Make sure your exhale lasts as long as your inhale. Repeat until you feel a sense of equilibrium, balance and calm beginning to return.

Attitude: Stay Young at Heart!

Good Karma

Give this quick karma trick a try. If you tell yourself that you'll get a good parking spot (and you really have to believe it), you will. If you say, "I'll never find a good spot," get ready to circle around for hours. It always works for me!

6. BAN NEGATIVE THOUGHTS

There's a positive and a negative side to every situation. Only you can decide which you would rather dwell on. You can complain about the rain or be thankful for the lush, green grass and well-nourished flowers. If you think you live under a black cloud, you probably will; likewise, if you anticipate positive outcomes, they'll be more apt to happen.

Everyone needs to vent once in a while—myself included. It isn't good to keep feelings all bottled up. But too much complaining can be counterproductive. It won't solve your problems. It won't help you lose weight. And it certainly won't help you turn back the clock.

Many of us aren't aware of our own negativity. Listen to yourself speak and try to become more conscious of it. Then practice turning those negative thoughts into positive ones. This isn't always going to be easy. There will be times that you'll just feel like sulking and complaining. But try not to do it. Remember, allowing pessimistic thoughts to linger can put your health at risk!

Over the course of my life I've learned to rephrase the negatives—I'll give you some examples. Then I want you to write down some of your main beefs and try rephrasing them in an optimistic light. This is a great mental exercise to do while you're walking or working out! Once you get the hang of putting a positive spin on negative feelings, it should start to happen automatically.

OLD NEGATIVE	NEW, POSITIVE APPROACH
My kids are driving me crazy.	My kids are smart, funny and talented—and they're a great excuse to exercise by running around the playground or going for a bike ride. It's also a great way to tire them out!
I'm fat.	I'm Rubenesque, beautiful and on my way to a healthy new body.

I can't do anything right.	No one's perfect, and I'm doing the best that I can. I prefer to focus on my achievements rather than my failures.
Nobody ever listens to me.	I'm in control and I'm going to make myself heard. If they didn't see me before, they will now!
If it's not one thing, it's another.	Life is full of challenges, and with a little ingenuity, I can successfully tackle each one.
I'm stuck in line, *again.*	I'm not going to get angry about things I can't control. Instead, I'll take this opportunity to Fidgetcize! Should I do calf raises or invisible butt squeezes?
I'm too old.	I'm just getting started.
I'll never look younger.	I may look older, but I'm also wiser.
It's not appropriate for my age.	Who cares! It's more fun to be silly than to be stodgy and boring.

_____   _____

_____

_____

_____   _____

_____

_____

_____   _____

_____

As soon as you notice pessimistic thoughts popping into your head, quash them immediately. Try putting a rubber band around your wrist and snap it whenever you find yourself being negative or critical. That's my favorite trick for instantly snapping out of it!

7. KEEP LEARNING

Youth is all about growth and learning. As children, we seemed to have countless hours to practice the piano, perfect our French accent or read the classics. But now that we're grown-ups we usually spend our free time paying bills, cleaning the house or watching TV.

Just because you're getting older doesn't mean that you should close the door on education experiences. Like all the muscles in your body, your mind needs regular exercise. So as you work to get your body in better shape, consider how to keep your brain stimulated. The advent of television has made it easy for us to spend free time zoning out in front of the tube. And while there are some rewarding TV programs out there, the majority of them aren't exactly stimulating.

You're never too old to learn, so find ways to keep your mind sharp and yourself interesting. Check out your community college for courses. Study while saving up for a trip to Italy. Take up a new hobby—painting or pottery or jewelry making. Read one worthwhile book a month or form a book club to discuss Oprah's favorites. (These are also great ways to expand your circle of friends.)

8. DON'T TAKE THINGS PERSONALLY

There's one woman in my neighborhood who has a way of making people feel bad about themselves. One night at a party she said to me, "Oh, Denise, sometimes when I see you, you look really good, and other times you look really chunky." My girlfriends who overheard the comment were shocked—how could she be so unbelievably rude? But I know that she often makes insensitive remarks like that to everyone, so I was able to laugh it off.

Other people are going to say and do things that hurt your feelings, either out of jealousy or stupidity or (sometimes) because they had a little too much to drink. I know it sounds clichéd, but it isn't you, it's them. People usually say mean things out of insecurity or unhappiness. So rather than waste your time wondering what's wrong with you, try to shrug it off and, if you can, steer clear of that person for a little while.

By refusing to see yourself as a victim, you'll be less likely to suffer the negative effects of someone else's insensitive or rude behavior. If you do start to feel upset or angry, take a few deep breaths or go for a walk—it'll help calm you down. Whatever happens, don't stoop to their level. Always be the bigger person—and don't lose your sense of humor!

9. LIE ABOUT YOUR AGE— AT LEAST TO YOURSELF

I'm not suggesting that there's anything wrong with looking your age or proudly celebrating your 50th birthday. But some women use their age as an excuse to slow down and stop trying. "I'm too old to take up skiing." "A person my age shouldn't go in-line skating." "You can't teach an old dog new tricks." Forget it! The minute you stop getting out there and challenging yourself, you start turning into that "old dog."

Pretending that you're 10 years younger—even if it's just in your own head—can help eliminate those old-age excuses that may be holding you back. Maybe you can't imagine trying rock climbing, saving up for a hiking trip to Nepal or sleeping in a tent at your age. But what if you were in your 20s or 30s? Why not? You have nothing to lose—and lots of rich, meaningful experiences to gain.

If you've always been the kind of person who plays it safe, it's never too late to learn to develop a sense of adventure. Some of the greatest rewards in life include some measure of risk. You're the only one who loses if you're unwilling to step outside of your comfort zone. Don't let your desire to be comfortable outweigh your desire to live a full, vibrant life!

10. LAUGH AND HAVE FUN

There is nothing like fun and laughter to get you through the tough times and to remind you of the joy that surrounds you. So take time to be silly—tell jokes, throw a Frisbee, fly a kite or pay the toll for the person in the car behind you. Try to have at least one good belly laugh every day. All this play is powerful: Many experts say that it can boost your immune system and help keep your body disease-free.

You're not the only one who will benefit from a little lightheartedness. So will everyone around you—from your kids to your parents to the guy who sells you a bottle of water each morning. Smile and you are guaranteed to get a smile in return. Enthusiasm is infectious. Happiness and a positive attitude are gifts you can pass along—so get out there and start giving!

Pleasure does more than make you feel good— it's good for you! Experiencing pleasure can boost your immune system for up to two days, so get out there and have fun!

YOUR 28-DAY CHALLENGE

Time to decide what you're going to work on in terms of attitude for the next four weeks. Think about what aspects of your emotional life could

Attitude: Stay Young at Heart!

use a tune-up. Do you need to practice some positive self-talk to improve your self-image? Should you figure out how to streamline your life so you don't get so stressed out? Is it time for you to reevaluate your friendships and start putting more energy into the ones that make you happy? Make your mental list, then write down your goals here:

Week 1: _____

_____

_____

_____

Week 2: _____

_____

_____

_____

Week 3: _____

_____

_____

_____

Week 4: _____

_____

_____

_____

Now get out there and think positive!

8

The Power of the Pyramid

Now that you've finished reading about all five levels of the Anti-Aging Pyramid, you may be excited to start making positive changes. You're ready to shed that excess weight, firm up those jiggly muscles, regain your energy and protect your body from illness. Or maybe you're feeling a little overwhelmed—you have so many changes to make that you're not sure where to begin.

While you might have the enthusiasm and motivation to immediately change every aspect of your life (and I'm glad that you do!), I want you to succeed. So before jumping in, take a few minutes to plot your course for the weeks ahead. You already know my formula for turning back the clock. Now it's time to figure out the best way for you to put this plan into action.

If you've read this book from cover to cover, you may already have determined your goals for the next four weeks. If not, do it now. At the end of each section you'll find a place to write down these goals—your 28-Day Challenge. For each level of the pyramid you should have four short-term goals. Instead of trying to master all of these goals at once, you'll focus on one goal from each section of the pyramid per week. Based on my experience, this kind of slow, controlled approach is the key to making those healthy habits stick. Think of it as training your body and mind in habits that will last *forever*.

When you're setting your goals for the next four weeks, remember to keep them small and achievable. Consider each one a stepping-stone toward your ultimate, long-term goal. For example, your long-term goal may be to fit into a size 12, but your immediate goal may be to do four cardio workouts per week or stop eating candy. To keep yourself from getting bored or losing motivation, continue challenging yourself by periodically updating your goals. I set new goals for myself at the start of each month—anything from learning a new yoga pose to reading a good book. Turning back the clock means staying ahead of the game, so you must constantly focus on *moving forward.*

Remember trying to learn how to play the piano or speak a foreign language as a kid? Repetition and practice were essential to mastering new skills. Well, the same goes for developing good health habits. Whether you're trying to make deep breathing or wearing sunscreen part of your daily routine, you need to practice, practice, practice. It may be hard to get in the swing of these things at first, but keep plugging away and your efforts will pay off. You need to make your body a top priority and pour as much interest and energy into your health as you do into other activities.

Throughout this book I've talked a lot about looking younger. While concerns about your appearance may inspire you to lose weight or start exercising, they probably won't be enough to keep you motivated over time. So as you progress, try to focus on how your body feels versus how it looks. Do you have more energy? Can you walk up a flight of stairs without huffing and puffing? Are you calmer and less stressed? Do you find yourself seeing the bright side of things rather than dwelling on the negatives? Concentrate on feeling good, and a healthy, beautiful body should follow.

As I mentioned in the beginning, all five levels of my Anti-Aging Pyramid are interconnected. This should be more evident now that you've finished reading the book. If you smoke or skip meals, it will be harder to exercise. If you eat right and get enough sleep, you'll be energized for your workouts and your mood will be elevated. When you exercise, you sleep better and look more refreshed. A nutritious meal plan means glowing skin and shiny hair. You can't get by with just one piece of the pyramid—you need all five!

A healthy, happy life requires *balance.* These days women play many roles. We're career women as well as moms, wives, daughters, sisters and friends. On the job we're competing in a man's world, where it's almost impossible to sneak away to our own lives at five o'clock. It's easy to get stuck on the merry-go-round of life, moving too fast and never stopping. Meanwhile we're suffering bulging waistlines, headaches, exhaustion, mood swings and back pain. That's why we need to recognize the need for fulfillment in many areas of our lives and create balance ourselves.

Decide right now how you want the rest of your life to turn out. If you believe that you can have more than you do now, you will. Taking good care of your body will make you feel better about yourself. You'll be more energetic and productive. You'll be able to experience and enjoy all that life has to offer. You'll know that you're doing everything possible to preserve your health and live your dreams.

No matter what your age, it's not too late to turn your life around. Even if you've lived on cheeseburgers or smoked a pack a day for most of your adult life, you can undo some of the damage to your arteries and lungs by changing your habits now. You can lower your risk of heart disease and diabetes by eating right, exercising and losing weight. You can reverse bone loss by taking up strength training and boosting your calcium intake. But you shouldn't waste another moment getting started!

For some of you, making healthy changes to stay fit and fabulous after 40 will be easy. Others of you will struggle. Whenever you're having trouble, try the mental trick that I use whenever I'm on the verge of doing something unhealthy. For instance, if I'm tempted to eat a big dish of frozen yogurt or go outside without sunscreen, I ask myself, "Would I want my daughters to do this?" The answer is usually no, which puts things into perspective and serves as an excellent deterrent.

It's easy to put off making positive changes until tomorrow or the next day. But the longer you wait to ditch those bad habits, the less likely you are to do it. By delaying, you'll only create bigger problems for yourself and prolong the negative feelings that you have about your body. You'll miss out on opportunities for adventure that begin with taking charge of your life and your health.

Good health is more valuable than money. It's worth more than a fancy car or an expensive piece of jewelry. I'm not saying that it's wrong to want financial success and all of its rewards. But it shouldn't come at the cost of your physical health and spiritual well-being. After all, what good is it to be the richest person on the block if you're too sick or tired to enjoy it?

Putting your health and happiness higher on your agenda isn't selfish—it's better for everyone around you. If you're still feeling guilty about spending time on you, have an honest chat with yourself. Wouldn't your husband love to see you slimmer and healthier even if he has to give up homemade desserts? Wouldn't your kids be happy if you hiked and biked with them instead of keeping your house as clean as a Hollywood set? You'll be teaching them to take care of their bodies by your good example.

As you move forward I want you to notice and appreciate every one of your accomplishments. When you pass on the donuts during a breakfast meeting at work, give yourself a pat on the back and say, "That was easy, and I can do this!" Whether you complete your first 1-mile walk or conquer a 40-mile bike trip, note how good you feel afterward—and remember that feeling the next time you consider skipping a workout. Occasionally reward yourself with a nonedible treat such as a new exercise outfit or a bottle of shower gel. You deserve it!

Education and growth are essential to turning back the clock, so don't stop with this book! Arm yourself with as much knowledge about health, fitness and nutrition as possible. If you're online, check out my Web site (www.deniseaustin.com) for updates and ideas about getting and staying fit. There are many terrific magazines and newsletters that provide helpful information on health, fitness, nutrition and skin care. We live in the Information Age—use these tools to help you stay young and healthy both inside and out!

On these pages I've told you everything that I know about turning back the clock—well, almost everything. What are my other secrets? Walking barefoot on the beach, shoulder massages from Jeff, toenail-painting parties with my girls, giggling on the phone with my sisters, watching sappy movies, taking warm baths, a sprig of fresh mint in my iced tea, freshly squeezed orange juice, the smell of lilacs, laughing and making others happy. Never underestimate the healing power of those little things in life. As I've said before, the best things in life don't come with hefty price tags. Quite often they're free. You only live once, so get out there and live to the fullest!

Appendix: Extra Recipes

As a bonus, I've included twenty-nine healthy, delicious dishes—so you can feast fabulously after 40.

Breakfasts

FAST FIX

Fiber-full French Toast
Makes 1 serving

2 eggs
⅛ cup skim milk
Cinnamon
Cooking spray
2 slices preservative-free whole-wheat bread (I pick up my bread from a local baker, but you can always use presliced bread from the supermarket)
½ cup fresh peaches or other seasonal fruit
1 tablespoon strawberry jelly

In a small bowl, combine 1 whole egg and 1 egg white. Add skim milk and whisk. Sprinkle cinnamon into mixture. Continue to whisk until well mixed. Coat nonstick pan with cooking spray and heat over medium heat. Dip bread slices into egg mixture until both sides are coated. Place in hot pan and cook until brown, about 2 to 3 minutes per side. Top with fresh fruit and a little strawberry jelly. I usually triple this recipe on the weekends, since my kids are crazy about French toast!

FAST FIX

Get-Your-Veggies Omelet
Makes 1 serving

4 egg whites
2 tablespoons water
Cooking spray
1 tablespoon chopped green onion
2 tablespoons chopped tomato
½ cup fresh spinach (or ¼ cup cooked)
1 ounce skim Swiss cheese, shredded
2 tablespoons salsa

Whisk egg whites with water until frothy. Spray nonstick skillet with cooking spray and place over medium heat until hot. Add egg mixture and cook for 5 minutes or until eggs begin to set. Sprinkle egg mixture with green onion, chopped tomato, spinach and skim Swiss cheese. Cook for another 2 minutes or until cheese melts. Top with any kind of salsa.

I just love the taste of Swiss cheese and spinach in an omelet!

Ginger Spiced Carrot Muffins
Makes 12 mini-muffins

2 cups all-purpose flour, sifted
4 teaspoons baking powder
Dash of salt
1 tablespoon ground ginger
1 teaspoon cinnamon
⅓ cup brown sugar
1 egg
¾ cup skim milk
½ cup applesauce
⅓ cup oil
1 cup grated carrots
Cooking spray

Preheat oven to 400 degrees. Combine sifted flour, baking powder, salt, ground ginger, cinnamon and brown sugar. In a separate bowl, mix egg, milk, applesauce and oil. Add carrots to milk mixture and whisk lightly into the flour mix. (Don't overmix.) Coat a muffin pan with cooking spray, then fill cups two-thirds full with batter. Bake for 18 minutes, then reduce heat to 350 degrees and bake for 5 more minutes.

Green Chili and Turkey Sausage Scramble
Makes 2 servings

2 ounces turkey sausage (medium spice)
4 eggs
2 tablespoons chopped tomato
2 ounces roasted green chili strips
1 tablespoon green chopped onion
1 tablespoon chopped cilantro
2 ounces pepper jack cheese, shredded
Cooking spray

Cook sausage according to package directions, then cut into ½-inch-thick pieces. In a small bowl, beat eggs with a fork. Add chopped tomato, chili, green onion, cilantro and cheese. Spray a small pan with cooking spray. Place over medium heat and add egg mixture. Stir eggs until cooked through.

FAST FIX

Oh, What a Beautiful Morning! Muesli
Makes 1 serving

½ cup muesli
½ cup water
1 tablespoon nonfat milk
1 teaspoon honey or brown sugar
1 tablespoon ground flaxseed
¼ cup low-fat vanilla yogurt
¾ cup fresh blueberries, strawberries or raspberries (or frozen and thawed)

Cook or microwave muesli with water according to package directions. Add nonfat milk and sprinkle with honey or brown sugar. Top with ground flaxseed, vanilla yogurt and fresh berries. This is delicious with freshly squeezed orange or grapefruit juice.

Lunches

GREAT ENTERTAINING

Caribbean Blackened Tuna Tacos with Mango Salsa
Makes 4 servings

2 tablespoons Caribbean jerk seasoning
4 tablespoons blackening spice (available in most supermarkets)
2 pounds fresh tuna steak (use red snapper if you can't find fresh tuna)
1 cup sliced mango
1 cup sliced pineapple
1 small red onion, diced
2 Roma tomatoes, diced
½ bunch cilantro, chopped
2 jalapeno peppers, finely chopped
Juice of 1 lime
4 small, low-fat flour tortillas
½ cup iceberg lettuce, shredded

Mix jerk seasoning and blackening spice, then rub onto tuna steaks. Let tuna marinate for at least 20 minutes. In a small bowl, mix mango, pineapple, onion, tomatoes, cilantro, peppers and lime juice and refrigerate. Grill tuna until light brown (about 2 minutes each side). Cut tuna into strips and place on tortillas, then top with shredded lettuce and mango mixture.

Chilled-and-Grilled Mai Tai Shrimp with Mango Mustard
Makes 12 skewers (about 3 to 4 servings)

12 jumbo shrimp, peeled
12 bamboo skewers

Marinade:
½ cup rum
½ cup grenadine syrup
1 cup sweet-and-sour sauce
1 teaspoon salt

Mango mustard:
1 cup mango slices with juice
⅓ cup Dijon mustard
1 tablespoon rice vinegar
2 tablespoons brown sugar

Combine ingredients for marinade. Place peeled shrimp on skewer lengthwise (one shrimp per skewer). Pour marinade over skewers and let sit for 1 hour. Grill until shrimp is cooked, usually about 1 to 2 minutes on each side. Refrigerate for 30 minutes. In food processor, add all ingredients for mustard and combine thoroughly. Serve chilled shrimp with mustard. Aloha!

Denise's Favorite California Club
Makes 1 serving

2 slices preservative-free whole-grain bread
2 ounces turkey, sliced
1 ounce low-fat Monterey Jack cheese
3 slices fresh avocado
2 tablespoons salsa

Toast bread. Add turkey, cheese, avocado and salsa. One of my friends brings an avocado and salsa with her to work, then buys a deli sandwich and gives it a fresh twist.

Gobble-It-Up Turkey Burger
Makes 4 servings

1 pound extra-lean ground turkey
1 packet Lipton California Onion Soup or Dip Mix

4 cups mixed greens
4 tablespoons low-calorie salad dressing

Mix together the ground turkey and onion soup mix. Form turkey into 4 burgers. Fire up the grill or coat skillet with nonstick cooking spray. Cook for about 3 minutes per side, or until cooked through. Toss greens with salad dressing and place on 4 plates. Place the cooked burger on the salad. This is a super-quick, super-tasty lunch!

Grapefruit and Black Bean Salad
Makes 4 servings

My girlfriends love when I make this for a special lunch.

Lettuce leaves
2 Florida grapefruits, peeled, thinly sliced and seeded
1 15-ounce can black beans, rinsed and drained
1 medium cucumber, halved lengthwise and sliced
1 cup cubed papaya
2 ounces reduced-fat Monterey jack cheese, cut into ¼-inch cubes

Dressing:
½ cup frozen Florida grapefruit juice concentrate, thawed
¼ cup water
2 tablespoons fresh cilantro, snipped
3 tablespoons honey
¼ teaspoon ground cumin

Arrange lettuce leaves on four salad plates. Place grapefruit slices on plates. Arrange beans, cucumber and papaya in mounds on lettuce. Sprinkle with cheese.

For dressing, combine juice concentrate, water, cilantro, honey and cumin in a blender. Whir for about 1 minute. Drizzle dressing over salads.

GREAT ENTERTAINING
Grilled-and-Chilled Tofu Skewers in Citrus-Ginger-Soy Marinade
Makes 8 to 12 skewers (about 3 to 4 servings)

Marinade:
½ cup light soy sauce
½ cup Florida orange juice
2 tablespoons canola or peanut oil
2 tablespoons sesame oil
2 tablespoons fresh ginger, minced
Dash red-hot chili sauce

1 package firm tofu, drained
16 medium shiitake mushrooms, trimmed
1 large daikon radish, sliced
1 head bok choy

Combine soy sauce, orange juice, oils, ginger and chili sauce and whisk to emulsify. Slice tofu cake in half. Cover with half the marinade and let sit at room temperature for 1 hour, turning frequently. Wash and trim mushrooms. Scrub and trim daikon and slice into 1-inch pieces. Separate bok choy leaves, rinse and pat dry. Set aside. Slice white bok choy stems into 1-inch-thick pieces. Marinate mushrooms, daikon and bok choy stems in remaining marinade for 15 minutes. Slice marinated tofu into 1-inch cubes. Brush bok choy leaves with marinade. Fold the sides of each leaf in toward the middle and roll up. Thread folded leaves onto wooden skewers alternately with mushrooms, tofu, daikon and bok choy stems. Grill skewers for 12 to 15 minutes. Turn to cook all sides. Chill skewers for at least 30 minutes and serve.

GREAT ENTERTAINING
Low-Fat Spinach Salad with Hot Turkey Bacon Vinaigrette
Makes 4 servings

Vinaigrette:
½ cup sliced low-fat turkey bacon
2 cups fat-free Kraft Italian Vinaigrette

Sauté turkey bacon until slightly crisp. Add vinaigrette and simmer over low heat for about 3 minutes, allowing bacon flavor to infuse. Set aside.

Spinach Salad:
8 to 12 cups fresh flat-leaf spinach
4 hard-boiled eggs
8 tablespoons corn kernels (use canned or thawed frozen corn for convenience)
12 wafer-thin slices of red onion
4 tablespoons fat-free shredded cheddar cheese

Wash spinach and pat dry. Slice eggs in half and discard yolk. Chop remaining egg white. Place all ingredients in a bowl and add hot bacon vinaigrette. Toss and serve immediately.

FAST FIX
Trim-Down Tuna Salad
Makes 2 servings

1 can albacore white tuna packed in water
1 teaspoon balsamic vinegar
1 teaspoon red wine vinegar
1 hard-boiled egg (with or without yolk), chopped
1 tablespoon white or green onion, chopped
2 cups mixed greens (I like spinach, arugula and romaine)
1 tomato, sliced

Rinse and drain the tuna and place in a bowl. Add balsamic vinegar and red wine vinegar and mix. If the tuna seems too dry, add another dash of vinegar. Mix in egg and onion. Arrange greens and tomato slices on 2 plates and top with tuna mixture.

Dinners

Herb-Poached Salmon with Roasted Tomato Vinaigrette
Makes 2 servings

Roasted Tomato Vinaigrette:
6 ripe tomatoes, cored and seeded
1 slice red onion
1 tablespoon fresh garlic, chopped
1 tablespoon olive oil
1 teaspoon brown sugar
1 teaspoon salt
1½ tablespoons red wine vinegar
1 tablespoon chopped fresh parsley

Herb-Poached Salmon and Rice:
1 cup uncooked brown rice
1 teaspoon olive oil
1 cup water
½ cup white cooking wine
2 tablespoons lemon juice
2 bay leaves
1 sprig fresh rosemary
1 sprig fresh oregano
1 teaspoon salt
1 slice yellow onion
1 celery stalk
2 4-ounce salmon filets

To make vinaigrette: Preheat oven to 300 degrees. Place tomatoes and red onion on a rimmed cookie sheet or broiling pan. Roast for 5 minutes. Place roasted tomatoes, onion and all remaining ingredients into a food processor and blend thoroughly.

To make salmon and rice: Prepare rice according to package directions and set aside. Place olive oil, water, wine, lemon juice, bay leaves, rosemary, oregano, salt, yellow onion and celery in a large, shallow saucepan. Bring to a boil. Immediately reduce to a medium simmer. Place salmon in saucepan using a slotted spatula. Cook for about 7 minutes.

To serve: Carefully remove the salmon and place on brown rice. Top with Roasted Tomato Vinaigrette.

Caribbean Jerk–Spiced Pork Chops with Sweet Potatoes
Makes 4 servings

½ cup Caribbean jerk spice
4 6-ounce thin pork chops
3 large sweet potatoes or yams
½ cup water
2 tablespoons butter
2 tablespoons honey
2 teaspoons kosher salt
Cooking spray

Preheat oven to 350 degrees. Rub spice on pork chops and let sit for 1 hour. Cut sweet potatoes in half, lengthwise. Place cut side up on rimmed cookie sheet with ½ cup water. Bake for 30 to 40 minutes. Spoon out insides and mash thoroughly with butter, honey and salt. Reduce oven temperature to 300 degrees. Coat a nonstick skillet with cooking spray and heat. Sear pork chops for 1 minute on each side. Place in an oven-safe dish and bake for 12 to 15 minutes or until done. Serve hot with sweet potatoes on the side.

Jeff's Favorite Sweet Potatoes
Makes 4 to 6 servings

I'm lucky to be married to someone who will eat just about anything. Over the years, I've started serving more sweet potatoes (great source of vitamins A and B$_6$ for women over 40), and this is Jeff's all-time favorite version. And I get the antioxidants (beta-carotene) I need in my diet.

4 large sweet potatoes, scrubbed and rinsed
1 teaspoon grated orange rind
¼ teaspoon allspice
Salt and pepper
⅓ cup light brown sugar

2 tablespoons butter
1 tablespoon fresh lime juice
1 tablespoon Grand Marnier liqueur (optional)

Preheat the oven to 400 degrees. Bake the sweet potatoes on the oven rack for about 45 minutes. Remove and turn the oven down to 350 degrees. Once cooled, peel and slice potatoes. In a shallow baking dish, place one layer of potatoes. Top with half the orange rind, allspice, salt and pepper. Repeat layer of potatoes and top with remainder of spices.

In a small pan over low heat, combine the brown sugar, butter, lime juice and liqueur until sugar is dissolved. Pour over top of potatoes and bake for about 30 minutes, spooning the glaze over the potatoes once or twice.

Let cool slightly before serving.

Mandarin Orange Barbecued Chicken
Makes 4 servings

This recipe needs to be made the day ahead to ensure that all the flavors meld. Make it in advance for a party!

Barbecue Sauce:
1 28-ounce can whole peeled tomatoes
½ cup brown sugar
½ cup rice vinegar
1 6-ounce can mandarin orange slices and juice
1 teaspoon salt
¼ cup tomato paste
1 dried red chili
1 tablespoon crushed fresh garlic
1 bunch cilantro

1 tablespoon salt
1 teaspoon black pepper
2 bay leaves
3 tablespoons blackening spice
¼ cup brown sugar
4 skinless chicken breasts
1 tablespoon salt
1 teaspoon paprika
2 tablespoons Cajun or blackening spice

Night before: Combine the sauce ingredients in a small saucepan. Bring to a boil, then simmer for 20 minutes. Puree the sauce, then cook an additional 10 minutes. Refrigerate overnight.

Fill a large pot with water; add salt, black pepper, bay leaves, blackening spice and brown sugar. Bring to a boil, then reduce heat. Add chicken and simmer for 60 minutes. Strain and refrigerate overnight.

30 minutes before serving: Season cooked chicken with salt, paprika and Cajun spice. Heat a charcoal or gas grill to medium-high heat. Sear chicken breasts on both sides for one or two minutes. (This can also be done in a nonstick skillet.) Remove from heat. Brush chicken breasts with barbecue sauce and place in ovenproof dish. Bake in preheated 300-degree oven for about 15 minutes or until the juices run clear.

Remove from oven and brush with sauce once more before serving.

My Mom's California Chicken Salad
Makes 4 servings

My friends adore this salad, and they always ask for the recipe. I warn them that's it's not exactly low calorie. But it does have plenty of protein. I've been making this salad since Jeff and I first got married and over the years I've adjusted the ingredients a bit, to make it lower in fat and calories. I love to serve this for summer dinners on the patio.

4 chicken breasts, with skin and bone
1½ cups low-fat or light mayonnaise
⅓ cup low-fat milk
½ cup Heinz chili sauce
2 tablespoons horseradish
2 tablespoons capers
1 tablespoon Worcestershire sauce
Juice of one lemon
½ cup pitted chopped black olives
⅓ cup chopped scallions
4 stalks celery, chopped
Chopped sweet pickles and pimiento for garnish (optional)
1 head iceberg lettuce
Salt and pepper to taste

Fill a large saucepan with water. Bring to a boil. Simmer chicken breasts (skin on) in liquid over medium heat until cooked, about 30 minutes.

Remove chicken breasts to cool. Once cool, skin and bone the breasts and tear chicken into bite-size pieces. Refrigerate 3 hours.

Combine mayonnaise, milk, chili sauce, horseradish, capers, celery, Worcestershire sauce, lemon juice, olives and scallions. Refrigerate. (Ideally, this should be made several hours in advance of serving.)

In a large bowl, tear iceberg lettuce into pieces. Mix chicken with the dressing and stir well. Arrange on top of lettuce and garnish with chopped pickle and pimiento. Add salt and pepper to taste and serve.

Poached Seafood Salad with Lime-Cilantro Vinaigrette
Makes 2 servings

Lime-Cilantro Vinaigrette:
2 bunches cilantro, chopped
1 cup lime juice
½ cup white wine vinegar
¼ cup brown sugar
¼ cup honey
1 tablespoon fresh garlic, minced
1 teaspoon salt
3 tablespoons Dijon mustard
¾ cup olive oil

Poached Seafood:
3 cups water
1 cup lime juice
1 tablespoon fresh garlic
2 tablespoons kosher salt
½ cup white wine
3 bay leaves (optional)
2 tablespoons brown sugar
3 ounces fresh salmon, diced
8 shrimp
4 ounces halibut, sea bass or your favorite white fish
8 scallops

Salad:
5 ounces mixed greens
lemon, sliced

To make vinaigrette: In a large plastic container, puree cilantro, lime juice and vinegar with a hand emulsion blender (or use a regular Oster-izer blender). Add brown sugar, honey, garlic and salt. Puree until smooth. Add mustard, then slowly add olive oil, little by little, as you mix with the hand blender or a whisk.

To poach seafood: Mix together water, lime juice, garlic, salt, wine, bay leaves and brown sugar. Bring to a boil. Add seafood, reduce heat to a simmer and cook for about 2 minutes. Strain seafood from water and place in a bowl with ¼ cup Lime-Cilantro Vinaigrette. Cool in the refrigerator.

To make salad: In a large mixing bowl, toss the salad greens with ¼ to ½ cup of the vinaigrette. Reserve remaining vinagrette for later use. Place on a salad plate and top with the cooled, poached seafood. Garnish with lemon slices. This is especially refreshing during those hot summer months.

Risotto with Oven-Roasted Portobello Mushrooms
Makes 4 servings

Risotto:
¼ cup minced yellow onion
1 tablespoon olive oil
2 cups Arborio rice
3½ cups defatted chicken broth
½ cup soy sauce
Salt and pepper to taste
½ cup grated Parmesan cheese
1 teaspoon chopped parsley

Portobello marinade:
½ cup salad or olive oil
⅔ cup balsamic vinegar
2 teaspoons salt
1 teaspoon pepper
2 tablespoons minced garlic
2 tablespoons Italian seasoning
4 Portobello mushrooms

To make risotto: In a large nonstick pan, sauté minced onion in oil over medium heat until translucent; add Arborio rice and stir to coat. Add broth and soy sauce, a little at a time, stirring constantly with a wooden spoon. Cook until broth is absorbed and rice is al dente. Season with salt and pepper to taste, then add Parmesan cheese and parsley and stir.

To make marinade: Preheat oven to 350 degrees. Mix first six ingredients and marinate mushrooms for 10 minutes. Reserve marinade. Place mushrooms with trimmed stems up on a cookie sheet and bake for 5 to 7 minutes. (Mushrooms can be made ahead and reheated.)

To serve: Place a spoonful of risotto in the middle of a plate and add a roasted Portobello mushroom on top. Drizzle with a little of the reserved marinade and serve.

Spinach-and-Red-Pepper-Stuffed Chicken Breast on Lemon-Asparagus Couscous
Makes 2 servings

2 cups couscous
Cooking spray
½ cup sliced asparagus
2 cups water
½ tablespoon salt

½ cup lemon juice

2 tablespoons brown sugar

2 4-ounce boneless chicken breasts

½ cup red bell pepper, roasted, peeled and chopped

1 cup fresh chopped spinach leaves

¼ cup part-skim shredded mozzarella cheese

Salt and pepper to taste

½ cup flour

1 tablespoon granulated garlic or minced fresh garlic

1 tablespoon canola oil

Pour uncooked couscous into a bowl and spray with cooking spray. Mix thoroughly. Blanch asparagus in boiling water for 40 seconds. Drain and add to couscous. In a separate pot, boil 2 cups of water. Add salt, lemon juice and brown sugar to boiling water. Pour heated water mixture into the bowl of couscous and let sit for 5 to 7 minutes until water is absorbed.

Preheat oven to 350 degrees. Cut a pocket in the chicken breasts. Stuff with red pepper, spinach, mozzarella cheese, and salt and pepper to taste. Combine flour and garlic. Close pocket and roll chicken lightly in flour mixture. Heat oil in nonstick skillet, add chicken and cook until golden brown. Place browned chicken in oven and cook for 30 minutes, until juices run clear. Serve chicken on couscous and asparagus.

Summer Citrus Swordfish with Basil and Tomato
Makes 4 servings

One of my friends always gives me her home-grown basil, and I love making this dish for Jeff and the kids. It's easy, delicious and high in protein.

4 tablespoons olive oil

1 small bunch fresh basil, finely shredded

Juice of 1 lime

Salt and pepper to taste

1 pound swordfish, in 4 pieces

1 cup finely chopped shallots

½ tablespoon minced garlic

1 bay leaf

½ cup dry white wine

¼ cup fresh lemon juice

1 cup clam broth

2 tablespoons chopped ripe tomato

Mix 1 tablespoon olive oil, 2 tablespoons shredded basil, lime juice, and salt and pepper to taste. Rub swordfish with mixture and let marinate for several hours.

Preheat oven to 450 degrees.

Rub a bit of olive oil onto a sauté pan, heat over medium heat and sear the swordfish on both sides, taking care not to burn it. The fish should look like it has a mild tan! Remove from pan, place in oven-proof dish and bake for 5 to 8 minutes, depending on the thickness of your fish.

Meanwhile, heat remaining olive oil in a sauté pan and add shallots, garlic and bay leaf. Cook, stirring often, until shallots turn translucent. Pour in the wine and lemon juice and stir, scraping up the bits from the bottom of the pan. Let simmer until liquid has reduced by about a third. Remove the bay leaf, add clam broth and continue simmering for about 4 minutes, until liquid is reduced by half. Add tomato and remaining basil. Stir and remove from heat.

Place swordfish portions on 4 plates and divide the sauce among them.

Turkey Piccata
Makes 4 servings

I'm always looking for new ways to serve turkey. It's so low in calories and high in protein, but I don't always want to spend the time it takes to roast a whole bird. This is a fast, delicious, lighter version of the standard veal piccata, using lean turkey cutlets.

1½ pounds turkey breast cutlets
Salt and pepper to taste
⅓ cup all-purpose flour
2 tablespoons olive oil
½ cup dry white wine
⅓ cup lemon juice
1 lemon, thinly sliced
1 tablespoon butter
Fresh parsley

Pound turkey breasts between two sheet of wax paper until the cutlets are about ⅛ inch thick. Sprinkle with salt and pepper; dredge in flour, coating cutlets well. Shake off any excess.

In a large skillet, heat 1 tablespoon olive oil over high heat. When hot, slip in half the cutlets and sauté until golden and the juices are clear, about 1 minute per side. Transfer to a warm platter. Add remaining oil to the pan and cook the remaining cutlets. Remove turkey. Add wine, lemon juice and lemon slices to the pan and bring to a boil, stirring to scrape up the browned bits. Remove from heat; swirl in butter. Pour sauce over turkey cutlets and garnish with fresh parsley.

Vegetarian Lasagna
Makes 4 servings

4 potatoes, thinly sliced
3 cups nonfat milk
1 teaspoon kosher salt
2 12-ounce cans tomatoes with basil
1 cup ketchup
1 tablespoon granulated garlic
2 teaspoons dried oregano
1 tablespoon brown sugar
2 cups cottage cheese
1 cup grated low-fat mozzarella cheese
1 teaspoon salt
1 can artichoke hearts
1 5-ounce can sliced mushrooms
1 16-ounce bag frozen vegetable medley
Cooking spray

Preheat oven to 325 degrees. Cook potatoes in milk until soft and starchy (about 4 to 5 minutes). Add salt. In a separate saucepan, mix together tomatoes, ketchup, garlic, oregano and brown sugar. Simmer for 5 minutes, then remove from heat and puree. In a separate bowl, mix together cheeses and salt. Drain canned vegetables and defrost frozen vegetables. Mix together in a medium bowl. Coat a small bread loaf pan with cooking spray. Pour one 4-ounce ladle of tomato sauce in bottom. Next place a layer of potatoes, covering the bottom. Cover with ⅓ cup of cheese mix. Add a layer of vegetables. Continue layering potatoes, sauce, cheese and vegetables. Be sure to finish with a layer of potatoes and sauce. Cover with foil and cook for 30 minutes. Let cool 1 hour. Reheat to serve.

Cannellini and Herb Crostini Salad
Makes 4 servings

This a super source of cancer-fighting fiber—most women over 40 consume only half the recommended 20 to 35 grams a day. Cannellini (white beans) are also loaded with calcium.

1 can cannellini, rinsed and well drained
¼ cup chopped shallots
¼ cup chopped flat-leaf Italian parsley
1 tablespoon olive oil
1 tablespoon red wine vinegar
1 tablespoon chopped fresh sage

1 tablespoon chopped fresh basil
1 garlic clove, crushed
Salt and pepper
4 to 6 slices French or Italian bread

In a bowl, toss beans with shallots, parsley, olive oil, vinegar, sage, basil, garlic, salt and pepper. (This is even better if made several hours in advance, refrigerated and then allowed to return to room temperature.)

Toast bread; top with a spoonful of the white bean mixture.

My friends also love this with chopped fresh tomato.

Desserts

Fruit 'n' Honey Yogurt Sundae
Makes 1 serving

4 ounces low-fat vanilla yogurt
1 tablespoon honey
Splash lemon juice
1 tablespoon slivered almonds
1 cup mixed berries

Mix yogurt, honey, lemon juice and almonds. Serve over rinsed berries.

Grapefruit Gratin
Makes 2 servings

2 large Florida grapefruit
4 teaspoons honey
4 teaspoons light brown sugar

Remove peel, pith and seeds from 2 large grapefruit and section. Arrange sections in two small, shallow ovenproof dishes. Drizzle each with 2 teaspoons honey and sprinkle each with 2 teaspoons brown sugar. Broil 4 inches from heat until light golden, about 5 to 7 minutes; sugar should bubble but not burn.

Lemon Sundaes
Makes 4 servings

This is a neat trick I learned recently from a friend who took a cooking class. I think the lemons make a wonderful, colorful display in a glass dish, garnished with fresh mint sprigs. You can also substitute lemon sorbet for the ice cream and orange sherbet, for a clever palate cleanser between courses at a dinner party.

4 large lemons
Low-fat vanilla ice cream or frozen yogurt
Orange sherbet
Fresh mint

Cut the top 1 inch off each lemon; reserve tops. Trim bottom about ¼ inch, so lemon stands upright. Carve out the flesh and discard. Scrape inside of lemons clean with a sharp knife. With a small scooper or spoon, layer scoops of ice cream and sherbet in hollowed-out lemons. Cover with lemon tops and freeze until ready to serve. Garnish with fresh mint.

Peach Smoothie
Makes 1 serving

4 ounces lemon yogurt
4 ounces skim milk
½ cup frozen or fresh sliced peaches
½ cup Florida orange juice
¼ cup toasted wheat bran
3 ice cubes

Place all ingredients in an Osterizer blender and whip until smooth.

Index

Page numbers of illustrations appear in italics.

Defy gravity with this fabulous workout video from Denise Austin...

STAY HEALTHY, STRONG, SLIM AND FIT... NO MATTER WHAT YOUR AGE.

Increase your metabolism through aerobic exercise combined with toning exercises that work the entire body...

Fit & Fabulous at Any Age is the perfect combination to reshape and rejuvenate your body.

Includes 20 minutes of fat burning aerobics, 15 minutes of body firming/toning exercises, 10 minutes of stress and tension relieving exercises.

Denise Austin

$14.98 OR LESS

FIT & FABULOUS at any age

AVAILABLE WHERE VIDEOS ARE SOLD

ARTISAN
HOME ENTERTAINMENT